Ka

Care Across Cultures
By
Robin Fisher

Communicating well with our ethnic patients

"The biggest problem in communication is the illusion that it has taken place."

From Robin,

Standing in fellowship
in the work of the
Kingdom.

Published by New Generation Publishing in 2020

Copyright © Robin Fisher 2020

First Edition

The author asserts the moral right under the Copyright, Designs and Patents Act 1988 to be identified as the author of this work.

All Rights reserved. No part of this publication may be reproduced, stored in a retrieval system or transmitted, in any form or by any means without the prior consent of the author, nor be otherwise circulated in any form of binding or cover other than that which it is published and without a similar condition being imposed on the subsequent purchaser.

ISBN 978-1-80031-975-2

www.newgeneration-publishing.com

New Generation Publishing

Care Across Cultures

Contents

Foreword 5

Part 1 –When Things Go Well 9

Part 2 –When Things Go Wrong 19

- The Language Barrier 22
- The Relationship 24
- Culture 24
- Medicines 25
- Minor Illness 28
- The Family 30
- Abortion 32
- The Doctor as Authority Figure 34
- Power Encounters..35
- The NHS 36
- Private Medicine 39

Part 3 –More Customs and Barriers. 43

- The Veil...43
- The Handshake..50
- Body Language 51
- Nursing 53
- Shame 55
- Magic and the Occult 59

- Qat 63
- FGM. and Other Cultural Issues. 65
- Gender 68
- Life and Death 70
- War and Civil Disruption 71

Part 4 – But I'm Not British! 74
- Are We 'Cold'? 74
- Relationships v. Efficiency 75
- Saying 'No' 77
- We Are Devious 79
- Racism 80
- Doctor, Doctor… 83
- Nurse, Nurse 84
- Professional Colleagues 85
- Women 86
- Patients 86
- Ethos 87

Part 5 – What Can We Do About It? 89
- Starting Ahead of the Game 89
- Confidentiality 90
- Accessibility 91
- Education 92
- Evolution 94

- Frequent Consultation 95
- Trust 96
- The Moral High Ground.. 96
- The Professional High Ground.............................. 98
- The Anthropologist 99
- Anthropological Methods: 99
- Finding a Cultural Mentor................................... 103
- Get a Good Interpreter 104
- Visits 108
- Teamwork 110
- Conclusion... 111

Foreword

The National Health Service is a huge multicultural experiment. Made up of workers from all over the world, the politically correct posters and pictures we are exposed to hardly do justice to its colourful diversity. With migrant workers from other continents, refugees, workers from all over the European Union and the growth of ethnic communities within this country, it looks after the interests of an increasingly diverse population.

This can be bewildering for both 'incomers' and those already here. A doctor, British by birth, despairs of understanding a gipsy lady recently arrived from Slovakia. A physician from Pakistan, newly practising in the UK, scratches his head, finding the people here completely incomprehensible and not a little unfriendly. Yes, he speaks English alright, but no one told him how to understand these strange people.

So if you have had an encounter with someone from a different culture that has left you feeling that things have spiralled out of control and you have not really understood what is going on, if you and your team feel swamped and rather intimidated by a group of people who you find incomprehensible, then this little book might possibly be of help and encouragement.

I hope that *Care Across Cultures* will enable you to have happy patients, but I have another agenda, and it's just as important. I want to see happy doctors, nurses, midwives, health visitors, physiotherapists and cleaners. Too much stress and misery is being caused by cross-cultural and linguistic barriers. I want to see people enjoying their cross-cultural encounters and their multicultural environments.

I have worked across cultures and across languages most of my professional life, with varying degrees of confusion and even success. I have worked in three health services – in Africa, in the Middle East, and in the NHS – and I have served in an area in Birmingham where nearly all my clientele were of Asian heritage. I have been richly rewarded with some deep relationships and a special place in people's communities that comes with the job. And I have had a huge amount of fun. I have learned that cross-cultural practice can be immensely enjoyable and that it can work!

I have also, for a few hours, been admitted to a hospital in another country and barely escaped being 'defibrillated'. I have frequently been an advocate for expatriate people in the Middle East who have experienced hospital admissions, sometimes for very serious conditions. It has been borne in on me, rather forcibly, that to be at the mercy of doctors and hospitals, if you are from another culture can be to feel utterly lost, disorientated and terrified.

My perspective is mainly that of a GP and jobbing doctor, but I hope very much that what follows will be of help to nurses and all others who care for or have to work with 'patients'. If you are one of these, you must forgive me for using the term 'doctor' most of the time but that is where I am coming from.

I hope too, that although I am British, and Anglo Saxon 'native English' at that, this book will not be too 'Anglocentric'. As I have noted above, my perspective is not so much about the British understanding the rest, but about all of us understanding each other.

So, the first part of this book outlines why encounters can go well. We have a look at the features that make for good communication and harmony. In the second part, we look at the cultural factors that are at the root of dysfunctional encounters and that can cause much pain and distress to us and our patients. There is a part for men and women coming from abroad to work in the NHS, to help them navigate the strange culture that they find here. In the fourth part, I suggest some of the means we can employ to lessen our confusion and make our consultations more productive and happy.

The very last thing I want to do is to give offence when I make remarks about cultures. I have been intentionally vague about the origin of many of my observations and my experience is necessarily incomplete and hopelessly biased. I have worked abroad long enough to look at my own culture from outside and to find it far from perfect and often most worthy of criticism. Please remember that if you are upset at anything you might find in these pages.

I have kept this book short and I hope easy to read. References are minimal. If you are looking for something academic you have pulled the wrong book off the shelf!

A note on language

I have always hated the word 'patient' and have tried to avoid it – however, there often seems to be no escape; 'client' and 'customer' just don't seem right. 'Ethnic' is a very useful word and I use it in its modern sense to mean loosely those who come from other cultures than the British; linguistic purists please forgive. 'Heritage' (i.e., 'Asian Heritage') denotes those who are born in this country of first or second generation 'incomers' or immigrants, or have arrived here at a very early age. It's hard to find a word that describes those of us who have been here for generations. 'Natives' or 'aborigines' are obviously not appropriate, correct though they undoubtedly are. 'Native British' or 'Native English' seem to work best for what is a difficult task.

I have tried to be gender neutral so 'he' and 'she' are interchangeable.

'Doctor' I have mentioned. If you are a physio, nurse, optometrist, manager or cleaner, please forgive me and don't fling the book into a corner.

(Almost) all names of people have been changed.

Part 1 – When Things Go Well

It is Monday morning at Small Town Medical Practice. Dr Jones is starting her surgery. She looks at her computer and, after briefly doing a moment or two's homework on her next patient, goes to the waiting room.

"Mr Smith? Come along in!"

Mr Smith puts down the waiting room copy of the *Racing Times* and follows Dr Jones into her consulting room.

"It's me chest again, Doc. Always happens at this time of year." Mr Smith gives an explanatory cough.

"Umm…" says Dr Jones. "And how much are you smoking these days?"

"Don't start on that one again. You know how difficult it is. I'm down to fifteen, but I can't touch them with this chest."

"Let's have a listen," says Dr Jones, after some appropriate questions. She has a good listen with her stethoscope. She suggests that, as it hasn't gone onto his chest, Mr Smith might like to take a prescription home and wait for a day or two to see if he gets better on his own.

Mr Smith thinks this a good idea and suggests an antibiotic that seemed helpful last time. "I'll do the inhalations too," he said. Dr Jones gets the message that Mr Smith is not in the mood for further strictures on his smoking. After a moment or two of conversation, Mr Smith gets up to leave.

Dr Jones looks at his back as he disappears. There is a little notice between his shoulder blades. It reads:

'Happy Patient'

But wait a minute: there are two people in this encounter. Dr Jones pulls open a drawer in her desk and pulls out a slip of paper. She glances at it, it reads:

'Happy Doctor'

I want to look at the sort of thing that makes consultations and interactions unravel when we are working cross culturally, and I suggest a few things that we can do to make things easier and more enjoyable for both patents and those who care for them. But, before I do this, it is helpful to look at the encounter that goes well, such as the one we have just looked at, to have a look at the factors that enable us to leave each other with 'Happy Patient' and 'Happy Doctor' (or 'Happy Nurse', or 'Happy Occupational Therapist') notices on our backs.

I am not going to dig into the detail of what a 'good consultation' or 'good encounter' is.[i] It is enough to say that if both (or all) those present leave happy then it is likely to have been a good encounter. Dr Jones, if she is a responsible and conscientious doctor, is not going to be happy if she has not done her job well; her patient can leave happy with the consultation even if the outcomes are not as good as they would have hoped for.

As Dr Jones and Mr Smith are intelligent and occasionally reflective people, they will realise that the good encounter that they have both experienced did not just occur naturally. There are important factors that make it that way. They are, in fact, sitting on a figurative iceberg, the submerged part of which contains the foundation of their successful meeting.

They speak the same language

Yes, they share the same mother tongue, but also much more; they pick up the same inferences, the same tiny phrases, the silences even. They each know not only how to make themselves understood but how to communicate in a way that is finely tuned. Dr Jones picks up that Mr Smith is not in the mood to discuss his smoking habit just now and that to do so would be counter-productive, perhaps even mildly damaging their relationship. There are ways around the language barrier when a mother tongue is not shared, but often there are more misunderstandings when the language is imperfectly known than if it is not known at all. It is said that American GIs leaving Vietnam with brides who knew not a word of each other's language had happy relationships until their brides began to learn English. Then the problems began.

They have an ongoing relationship

These two have known each other as doctor and patient for some time. This means that consultations are shorter; the doctor does not have to introduce herself and things can be picked up where they left off. Moreover, they have what we have called the 'doctor-patient relationship'. The fact that they are doctor and patient subtly affects their friendship. If Mr Smith and Dr Jones should bump into each other at Tesco's there is an understanding that they will not discuss medical matters unless the doctor initiates the subject, which she may just do. This is far from the case in some cultures.

In Sudan, I would often bump into patients in the street, whereupon their naturally smiling faces would crumple, they would clutch their stomach, doubling over in seeming agony. Many people just could not get over the fact that I was a doctor and here I was, in the street and readily available! This can happen with complete strangers as well, and airports seem to be predisposed to this.

I proffered my passport to a lady official at Khartoum airport who immediately burst into tears. It turned out that her mother was just starting her TB treatment and she urgently needed some reassurance. At Damascus airport, I had a stethoscope in my hand luggage. This meant that a customs officer and a rapidly growing bunch of his colleagues required advice on more and more complex matters; all of it free at the point of delivery. I only escaped by suggesting light-heartedly that all those requiring advice strip naked on the customs bench for examination.

In the UK we generally keep medical matters to the surgery and this supports and protects the relationship. But other cultures may have no such barriers. An understanding of this helps to reduce the stress and we are less likely to judge an individual for perceived rudeness.

They are in the same culture

Dr Jones and Mr Smith come from the same town and share a vast number of values and assumptions, which is something we need to look at. This makes for much better understanding. As we shall see, any or all of these values may not be shared if we are working cross culturally. Part of this is a shared history, and a shared view of it as well.

They understand what a GP is supposed to do

Dr Jones has a pretty clear idea of what she can do and what she should do, both as an individual and as what people see as 'a GP'. Mr Smith also has an idea of what Dr Jones should be able to do, and very importantly they coincide – not exactly, but to a great extent. In the scenario that we have looked at, both parties are sure that Mr Smith's cough is the proper province of Dr Jones. Dr Jones will be relieved that of all the difficult problems she will encounter that morning Mr Smith's chest will probably be the easiest; it will be a little light relief in between more intractable troubles. Very importantly, there is a shared view of who makes the decision to prescribe a medicine or not, and what it should be. In many cultures this is far from the case.

They have a shared view of minor illness

British people and those born in the UK are familiar with the concept that a 'cold', viral illness, or a 'tummy ache' is not something that the doctor can deal with and is possibly a waste of the doctor's time. These messages are reinforced by notices on the walls of waiting rooms. This concept is far from universal and requires a sophisticated awareness on the part of patients as to what may be serious and what may be trivial, and the time it takes to work out which is which. If Mr Smith had started to cough a couple of hours before it is likely that Dr Jones might have been inwardly slightly annoyed (she would never, of course, let Mr Smith see this!) as she would not be able to make a proper assessment of his chest at such an early stage and the cough might well have got better on its own. Mr Smith comes just at the right moment, which is a product of his knowledge of his own illness and his awareness of what a 'minor illness' is. We shall see that this awareness is often absent in those of other cultures and for good reason.

They have a shared understanding of why people go to the doctor

Tracy came to see me with her little boy of about a year old. "He's been coughing doctor," she said. "Can you check him over?" I did so and she stood up to leave. "Thanks, Doctor," she said, "I just wanted to make sure."

I was taken aback by the sheer simplicity of the encounter. She had really wanted exactly what she said and no more. When she had finished, she upped and left.

Mr Smith came to see Dr Jones for exactly the reason he says, and that makes the consultation straightforward with few hidden agendas. Moreover, there is a shared understanding of what a 'medical consultation' actually is, how long it should take, what should go on during it, and hopefully, how it should end. This is often not the case in different cultures, as we will see later on.

They understand what can and cannot be expected of the NHS

The NHS is a huge and complex organisation that is continually evolving and changing. Mr Smith and those of us born in the UK have a fairly clear understanding, or at least a working knowledge, of what the NHS is capable of, what is legitimate to ask of it, and what is impossible. What Mr Smith comes to see Dr Jones about is not only within the competence of a GP but is within the abilities of the health service. Mr Smith assumes that he will get his medicine and get it free and he is not disappointed. Furthermore, he will be aware of the kinds of operation that are available should he need one, the kind of hospital care that is available and the kind of things he should *not* be asking for. Dr Jones shares these assumptions about the NHS and here is another basis for their mutual understanding.

They have a shared folk lore about medicine

Most doctors are aware that their practice of medicine is, at times, rather closer to magic than they might like. In our UK culture we share various folk beliefs about health and disease; people catch colds from being in the cold; feeding people up makes them better. If I have a high temperature, I need to be kept warm. 'Trapped wind', 'gastric flu', 'a chill', and other conditions are not really recognised by medical science, but Dr Jones will be aware of what these expressions mean. There are many other beliefs, some innocuous, some harmful, and Dr Jones and Mr Smith are aware of these. Dr Jones will assume that most of these are ill founded and Mr Smith, without thinking about them very much, assumes they are more or less true. The important thing is that they both know about the sort of thing that the other person is talking and thinking about. When we work cross culturally, we may be quite unaware of important beliefs about health, disease and life generally, that are entirely different from our own and that will affect our patients' understanding of their condition and our understanding of our patients.

They have a shared view about confidentiality

Dr Jones may ask Mr Smith how his wife is, especially as she might have recently consulted her, or have some health problem, but she will be very aware of her professional ethic about confidentiality – where this can be relaxed a little, and where it needs to be strongly abided by. Mr Smith might ring up the surgery for his wife's test results but beyond that there will be – and should be – minimal sharing of information.

Both doctor and patient have a clear understanding of where the boundaries lie and harmony reigns when these are not transgressed. Of course, a vast amount of what goes on in a consultation is mundane and boring, but there is a special trust between doctor and patient when the latter understands that personal, embarrassing and compromising matters are held in trust and will go nowhere. We shall see that other cultures have entirely different ideas of what the doctor should tell them about other people.

They negotiate

There has been a quite rapid change in the way doctors persuade people to do what they think they should do. Words such as 'compliance' and 'concordance' spring to mind. Doctors used to tell their patients what they should do and they would expect them to get on with it with minimal explanation. I remember as a child seeing a hospital nurse striding by with patient notes under her arm. Emblazoned on the front in huge letters was 'NOT TO BE HANDLED BY THE PATIENT'. Those days are hopefully gone forever and we can see that Dr Jones and Mr Smith negotiate. They discuss what should be done. Dr Jones makes a suggestion and Mr Smith agrees, or perhaps disagrees and then there is a discussion. He thus, hopefully 'owns' the decision as to what should be done and maybe is more likely to carry it out. He is very happy to negotiate in this way and finds it perfectly normal. If there is a more complex matter, Mr Smith will expect Dr Jones to suggest some kind of plan, so that he knows what to expect over the coming period. And he expects to have some explanation in non-medical language that he can understand.

When I outlined this to Jordanian medical students, they were horrified. "People will not think we are proper doctors," they would say. "People expect us to tell them what to do; if we don't, they will think we don't really know what we are doing!"

Conclusion

Harmonious understanding and good communication rests on many assumptions: language, relationships, confidentiality, what doctors and the health service can and cannot do, who decides if a medicine is appropriate, how to negotiate plans and treatment. When these assumptions are unfounded trouble ensues.

Part 2 – When Things Go Wrong

Over to Big Town Medical Practice. Dr Rosina is the new trainee... she is from Asian heritage and was born in England.

Zofi is from Eastern Europe, from a Gypsy family. She has five children and here she is with her little baby boy, Jaromil. The family have just arrived in the UK and are living in Big Town in an overcrowded house in poor condition.

Dr Rosina. (*Goes into the waiting room*) Zofi and Jaromil Nemec? Hello! I'm Dr Rosina. Come along in, Lovely to see you! Welcome!

(*Zofi comes in with several children and three other family members*)

Zofi. My baby coughing. It is very terrible. He coughing all night and no sleeping. My husband he say take him to doctor and get him injection. He need cough mixture, and he need antibiotics. My husband say you fix him. You give him good medicine.

Dr R. (*Rather uncertainly*) Umm... yes, now let's start at the beginning... May I ask you a few questions first? How long has little Jaromil been coughing?

Z. Last night he starts. He barking like a horse. Listen to him. (*The baby doesn't make a sound*). He need medicine now, Doctor. (*The relatives murmur in agreement*).

Dr R. Yes… well, he doesn't seem to be coughing at the moment… Do you think he has a temperature? (*Feeling the baby*) He doesn't seem to have one now…

Z. He very hot in the night, Doctor. He coughing too bad. He need antibiotic.

Dr R. Well, yes… but he has only been coughing for a very short time… has he been eating well today? And drinking?

Z. He sleeping too much now. He eating and drinking milk OK… I help him drink milk. I put sugar in the bottle. Doctor, he need good medicine. I speak to my mother on the phone. She say take him to the doctor and get good medicine. English doctor will give medicine…

Dr R. Yes… er… What would happen at home if you took him to the doctor there?

Z. Doctor Konstantin he give good medicine. He very good doctor. If I pay he give injection, he give vitamins and maybe many medicines. Here medicines good and free!

Dr R. Maybe I can just have a look at little Jaromil. *(She makes a show of examining Jaromil carefully)* What I would like to do is wait for a day or two; this is probably a virus and it will get better on its own…

Z. *(Upset, confused and getting a bit panicky)* But doctor he very sick. He got diarrhoea and vomiting, he need medicine.

Dr R. *(Feels rightly that she is losing control)* Well, Jaromil seems to be in pretty good condition at the moment...

Z. *(Unimpressed and interrupts)* Doctor, my sister back home, she needs medicine for her back...She very pain too much. You give me medicine for her.

Dr R. I am really sorry but we can't give medicine unless we actually see your sister. I might give her quite the wrong medicine if I haven't examined her...

Z. You no good doctor! You no give medicine! All doctor give medicine!

(Z gets up and leaves, her family troop out, obviously unhappy and unsatisfied.)

As Zofi goes, Dr Rosina sees something we have all seen. Tucked neatly between Zofi's shoulder blades is this notice:

'Unhappy Patient'

Dr Rosina pulls open the drawer of her desk and, just as her colleague Dr Jones has done, she pulls out a notice. On it is written is:

'Unhappy Doctor'

Yes. Dr Rosina is really unhappy. It has been a rotten consultation; Zofi and her relatives were obviously cross and dissatisfied and confused. Dr Rosina goes to the loo to have a quick cry.

What has gone wrong?

This situation may seem exaggerated and far-fetched but I promise you that I have heard every sentence many times. And felt just as Dr Rosina feels. The consultation is just the opposite of what has occurred in Small Town. Instead of harmony, there is conflict. Instead of a clear progression to a desired end, there is dysfunction. Instead of each participant in the encounter feeling secure in knowing where the event is going, there is confusion and uncertainty.

Why has it all gone so badly wrong?

- **The Language Barrier**

It is obvious that Zofi does not speak English well. She makes herself understood but she is having an uphill struggle from the start. As I said earlier, real difficulties emerge when your patient starts to speak English. You will immediately say to yourself 'She Speaks English' and greatly overestimate her powers of both comprehension and expression. She is able to state a few facts but that is about it. When trouble starts, things quickly fall apart.

Moreover, it is possible that Zofi is unable to read English. It is even more likely that many women first generation incomers from the Indian subcontinent, the Arabian peninsula and refugees from parts of Africa will be illiterate in their own mother tongue. I have asked many of these ladies in my own practice how much education they have received. Nearly all had two years of primary education or less. Some had none at all. They are not well equipped to learn another language and another script. It is well established that maternal literacy is a key factor in child health. If a woman cannot read, the deluge of print that we subject our patients to; the appointments, reminders, texts, and health promotion leaflets are all entirely pointless. Yet we cannot *see* that a person cannot read, and people quickly become afraid to admit it. Nevertheless it is a crucial factor in a woman's own health and the health of her family. This is nothing to do with intelligence. It is nearly all due to lack of opportunity.

Rosina, for her part, probably speaks an Indian or Pakistani language, such as Urdu or Punjabi, but all her schooling has been in English and this is her functional best language and she is just as at ease in it as her native English friends.

"Three days no she toilet" or "This my knee too much pain" underline the fact that a complete lack of grammar will get you a long way, but we soon find that when it comes to mental illness or the subtleties of a normal healthy consultation, we are in the dark. I spent many hours learning Urdu, the national *'lingua franca'* of the Asian people of central Birmingham. This did wonders for my relationships and was seen as a sincere attempt to get close to people. However, all I succeeded in doing was convincing my clientele that I spoke their language far better than I really did, leading to yet more misunderstanding as well as much laughter. To make matters worse, I discovered that, although many people understood my basic Urdu, they replied to me in yet another language, their mother tongue, and a tribal dialect.

- **The Relationship**

We all have to start somewhere, but this encounter with Zofi and her family has been a terrible beginning. The relationship is foundational to the consultation; even if there is no history, there needs to be a degree of rapport. Our relationship difficulties can be overcome by an understanding of the factors that make this encounter difficult and by seeing relationships in the long term. This is not just a consultation, it is a relationship that can be painful or rewarding, productive or ineffective, in the future if it is handled rightly. And the doctor is the one who needs to be informed enough to guide the relationship into something that can be enjoyed by both.

- **Culture**

In the scenario above Zofi is at a severe disadvantage. She has come to a culture where all the goal posts are in different places. She is not really aware of this, just that things are turning out in a way she did not expect, and she cannot understand why, one by one, her needs are not being met. If you are encountering a refugee family from the Middle East, or a young migrant man from Africa, the same confusion is likely to prevail. Much of what follows can be seen as cultural difference. Of course, we don't *see* the difference and that is part of the problem.

In our own culture we expect so much; we swim in a sea of familiarity, of sounds, people, situations, behaviour, that we know and interpret correctly. Zofi, and people like her, are swimming in a sea that is full of the strange and the incomprehensible. Worse, she thinks things are comprehensible and is confused; she looks at a situation that is familiar in her home context but is actually quite different here. she thinks that a doctor's appointment should be the same as in her home country – but it isn't!

- **Medicines**

Zofi comes from a culture where the patient, not the doctor, decides that they should get a medicine. This is quite fundamental to many cultures all over the Middle East and Africa. When I was training primary health care workers in Sudan, I realised on day one that the advice you would give to a trainee doctor in the UK just would not do. The British GP expects to decide whether his patient needs a medicine or not – this may involve some negotiation but the patient will usually accept that this is within the sphere of what the doctor does.

This is far from the case in Africa or the Middle East. If the patient has made the effort to see a health professional – and this may mean travel, expense, much time lost, and the entire family going – they have made the decision that they are to have a medicine, preferably several, maybe four or five, and preferably by injection. It is part of the contract. One could almost describe a doctor as 'one who gives medicines'.

"...But if I don't give a medicine they will say I am not a proper doctor," the medical assistant in Sudan would say. Moreover, she probably thinks, 'And I won't *be* a proper doctor'.

In a mission hospital in Yemen the clinic helper takes me outside into a secluded place. "You aren't giving enough medicines!" he remonstrates. "This lady has come fourteen miles. She and her family walked all night; and you gave her only two medicines – and no injections! You must give five medicines," he says, thrusting his palm at me, all five fingers outstretched. "*Five!*"

In Port Sudan, I was on a visit with my wife to a family of nomads. As we got up to leave, a delegation came from next door. Would I please look at the baby who is very sick?

Very foolishly, I agreed. I went over to look at the baby, who seemed fine. I made a great show of listening to the mother and family, and of examining the child very carefully. In the end, I suggested that there was not a lot wrong, but as I was passing that way in the morning I would call and have a look at the baby again. There! I had indicated in every way that I cared a lot and had made every effort.

In the morning, I called as promised. The evening after I left, the baby had been taken to a 'proper doctor', it had received what every child in Sudan receives from every doctor: an anti-malarial, an antipyretic and an antibiotic. The child was none the worse for this routine polypharmacy but I was mortified and learned my lesson. All my non-verbal signals that I was taking the greatest care were completely wide of the mark. My failure to give a prescription was seen as neglect.

Back in Birmingham, Shagufta, a young Asian mother, brings her little Asif to the surgery. He has a temperature. Shagufta is full of insight into her own culture. I start to give her some careful advice, saying that Asif doesn't really need an antibiotic, but I would gladly see him again tomorrow if she felt it was necessary.

"Thanks, Doc," she replies. "That's great, but this isn't good enough for my mum-in-law. She will get really upset if I don't bring back a bottle of something. Look… I promise to do all the things you say and I won't use the medicine, but can you just give me a prescription to keep my family quiet?"

Shagufta has understood the problem precisely! The older members of the family are first generation immigrants and their culture says that a doctor gives medicine, otherwise he is not a proper doctor. Moreover, the baby will definitely not get well without it. Maybe we should change our doctor to a better one?

In our scenario, Zofi is genuinely confused and upset by Dr Rosina's inability or unwillingness to give her a medicine for her child. Is she not a real doctor? So desperate is she to wring a prescription out of the doctor that she changes tack entirely and starts to talk of little Zaromir's diarrhoea, previously unmentioned, in the hope that this will get her a medicine.

It goes further. Dr Rosina examines little Jaromil very thoroughly. She is trying to communicate non-verbally that she is exercising great care over the little boy. This is her body language. But it is all wasted on Zofi and her relatives. The language of care is how many medicines you give. However carefully I communicated to the nomad family that I was taking the utmost care, my efforts were wasted. The giving of medicines is what communicates care.

If a doctor understands her patient's cultural attitude to medicines, she will be in a better position to understand and not judge.

- **Minor illness**

Dr Rosina looks at little Jaromil. In her mind, something like this goes on. "A cough? A few hours? Surely she knows that kids get this sort of thing all the time? This is a wasted consultation!" She feels a bit miffed.

But this is not justified. In Western Europe and the UK we have sophisticated and readily accessible health services. Child mortality is very low. There is a high standard of environmental health. Rubbish is collected, water is clean. We can afford to be a bit relaxed about our children's health.

But in many countries this is far from the case. In many parts of Africa and Asia, the infant mortality rate is high. There may be a patchy immunisation programme, or none at all. The water is polluted and there is a constant risk of diarrhoea. Malnutrition means that children are less able to resist the onslaught of illnesses that have virtually disappeared in the West. Parents know that their children are at risk in the first few years of life and there is often a high level of anxiety. Furthermore, in very hot climates, a high fever or an episode of vomiting can lead to dehydration and collapse within an hour or two. In this situation, 'wait and see' is madness and can be fatal. Added to this, some of our patients will have come from conflict areas where keeping children safe and well fed – or fed at all – is a moment by moment struggle.

Many of our ethnic patients will have this as their background. Furthermore, the 'minor illnesses' themselves present differently. Children in the Middle East and Africa are much more likely to get fevers or diarrhoea than 'snuffles'.

It takes time for people to understand the prevailing health environment. Shagufta above has learned about minor illness, but her parents-in-law and older family members are still in the mindset of their home country. In our practice in Birmingham we saw the children all the time. It was immensely hard work but slowly parents began to understand that children did not need to be seen at every snuffle or cough. This was far from the solution to our very high attendance rates, as there were other reasons why people came to the doctor, as we shall see. Zofi may, in time, be a little more relaxed about bringing Jaromil to the surgery, but this may not in itself reduce her attendances as there are other powerful forces dictating whether she comes to the doctor or not, as we shall see.

- **The Family**

Most of the time, in our own country, people decide to visit the doctor when they are unwell and, broadly speaking, we reckon that they make the decision themselves. In our very individualistic society, there is some truth in this. Parents obviously decide to bring their kids. Men are reckoned to be very reluctant to visit the doctor and sometimes a man's wife will come too. Figuratively, she has a pistol in her hand and he is there at gunpoint. But, in our first scenario, there is no suggestion that Mr Smith's decision to see Dr Jones is made by anyone other than himself.

In the second scenario, it is different. We see Zofi coming in with three family members. It is at once clear that it is her husband who has decided that she should bring Jaromil to the doctor, but he himself is not present. Furthermore, he has decided the outcome in his absence and Zofi (and perhaps Dr Rosina) realises that he will lose face if the outcome is not as he has decreed. To complicate matters, Zofi's mother, back in her home country, has a hand in this as well – and so does her sister who wants something else entirely. Is this difficult for the doctor? Spare a thought for the poor patient who has to satisfy the agenda of all of them. Both Zofi herself and the doctor are under enormous pressure.

This is far from unusual. In many cultures, in Eastern Europe, the Middle East and Africa, it is the family who makes the decisions, the elder ones having the greater – or perhaps the only – say. That one person, and especially a younger person and a woman at that, should make a decision unilaterally is quite outside their cultural framework. In addition, we need to remember that, in a very large number of cases, marriages are arranged by the parents, which further alters the influence and power hierarchy. In countries I have worked in it is most unusual for people to attend the doctor alone. In Yemen, not less than ten or twelve people would come to the hospital. They would watch over the encounter closely to see that all was done properly.

I have often found myself at sea during a consultation, and wondering with mounting anxiety what was going on. Often the poor patient or their mother is trying to satisfy the agenda of half a dozen different people, most or all of them absent. Shagufta realises perfectly the situation she is in and is very skilful at coping with it. Others are not so fortunate or insightful. It could not be more different than my encounter with Tracy that I mentioned earlier. She had no family agenda and things seemed a lot simpler.

Who had asked – or told – a person to come to the surgery, and what they were expecting, was a question I got into the habit of asking. Very often it was a mother or mother-in-law, a husband or the whole family. Often a mother makes her decision to bring a child simply because she wants to indicate to her family that she is properly caring for him.

- **Abortion**

This family way of making decisions is thrown into sharp relief when there is a request for an abortion. Sabina was pregnant with her fourth child. She came with her husband requesting a termination of pregnancy. Sabina's husband did most of the talking and Sabina herself was unnaturally quiet.

I managed to persuade the couple to wait for a while as Sabina was only a few weeks pregnant. I saw them both two or three times and became more and more convinced that things were not right. Finally, I managed to see Sabina on her own. She broke down in tears and sobbed that she didn't want an abortion. Her husband and family had made the decision and she was powerless to resist.

With support for Sabina, and much negotiation, the family revised its decision. We held our breath and, in due time, Sabina came to the ante-natal clinic. We all rejoiced.

A few months later, I was walking down the street where Sabina and her family lived. There was a bellow from across the road and I saw Faisal, Sabina's husband, holding a little baby high above his head. He ran across the road and thanked me profusely for 'not allowing them to have an abortion'. That wasn't quite the way I saw it, but there was a happy outcome.

This underlines the family dynamic that makes arriving at decisions a corporate affair and contrasts sharply with the current emphasis on choice. A westernised young woman who is from an indigenous British background may have significant, perhaps total autonomy when it comes to making choices in her life, backed up by a strong belief in her personal ownership of her own body. She may request a termination and her doctor may assume that she is making a decision for herself.

A woman from an Asian culture will be in an entirely different position. As I have emphasised earlier, individual choice in important matters is unthinkable, and even her choice of marriage partner may have been very limited. A lady requesting an abortion may be under pressure from her family in just the way that Sabina was, and health workers need to be conscious of that possibility. This becomes more acute with relaxations in the law on abortion that we can expect in the near future, and the ability to determine the sex of the unborn child by scan and other means early in the pregnancy. The advent of tests to determine the sex of an unborn baby will render gender-linked abortion even more possible and likely in cultures where there is an extraordinarily high premium placed on male children.

There is mounting evidence that abortion on the grounds of gender is becoming more and more widespread worldwide and is becoming more common in Britain. As our indigenous culture fixates on the value of 'choice', we are surely witnessing a practice that strikes at the very heart of gender and sexual equality as well as the value of the unborn baby itself.

- **The doctor as authority figure**

Underlying much or all of this is the kind of relationship that the doctor and their patient assumes. There has been a marked cultural change in the way authority figures are viewed in Britain. This works through into the health sphere in that, as we have mentioned elsewhere, doctors and health staff are far more accountable than half a century ago. But this may not be so in countries where many incomers are from. Many of your patients will view your well-meant attempts to negotiate treatment plans as a sign of weakness and ignorance, and they might be much more confident when just told what to do!

In our own practice It was very noticeable that people from the subcontinent were in this category, where the doctor was essentially an authority figure; but most of their children had adopted the western perspective where they considered themselves entitled to be fully informed and consulted. As a junior doctor, I was clerking a lovely old lady. In the course of the examination, I noticed an enormous and very ancient scar on her abdomen.

"May I ask what this was for?" I asked.

"Well, no one ever told me."

"But you didn't ask?"

"I thought it was none of my business."

Hopefully those days and those attitudes have gone forever.

- **Power encounters**

It is frequently through the family dynamic that power encounters occur. Majid came with his sister and a cousin, who was a well-known paediatrician in another town. The sister had been suffering from chronic hip pain. It was at once clear that the paediatrician in the family needed to dictate events. He proceeded to outline what should be done and where. I understood that this attitude was necessary because of his high status as a doctor in the family. The problem was solved by us both stepping outside and agreeing that, should he wish to arrange things himself, he was at liberty to do so privately, and perhaps he should consider paying for this; but in the health service things work differently and, as the family had taken the trouble to come to see me, would he please agree to accept my judgment?

Regrettably, the surgery is often a place where power encounters are manifested and this can cause severe dysfunction. The surgery is absolutely not the place for these conflicts to be played out.

- **The NHS**

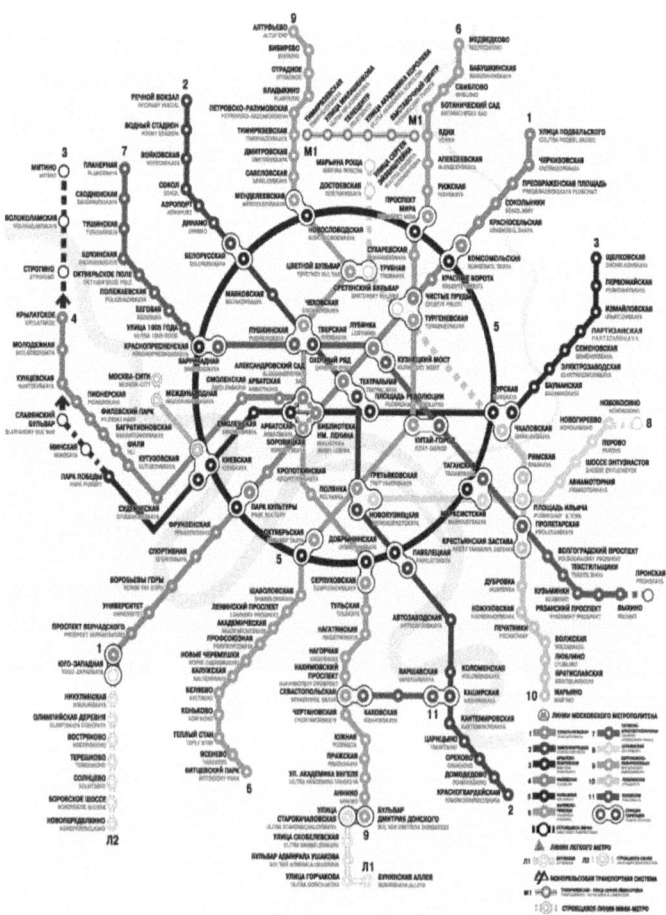

Map of the Moscow Metro

Come with me to the Moscow Metro. The place names are in Russian and you cannot read them unless you read Cyrillic script. If you get a Latin script version, you will get the illusion that you understand it and you will launch out, with dire results. You may think it bears some resemblance to the London Underground but once you get on to it you find that the crowds are overwhelming, the escalators are as long and precipitous as Olympic ski jumps, the announcements incomprehensible and the stations like cathedrals.

Now picture a person newly arrived in Britain. Someone has told them about the NHS, how it is all free, reliable and – above all – accessible. But their experience is going to be like mine on the Moscow underground. They will get lost.

As we saw in chapter one, Mr Jones and his family have a finely nuanced idea of what the NHS can provide and what they can ask of it. While younger generations that grew up when there was a welfare state tend to be rather more demanding, those brought up in the UK will have a clear idea of the complex and always changing nature of the health service.

But Zofi comes from an entirely different culture, where private medicine is paid for and the rules are different. Dr Konstantin, her doctor at home, provides many medicines when she asks and, for a small extra consideration, will provide an injection. Now she is in Britain, medicines – and presumably injections as well – are free, but she isn't going to get any! The goal posts have moved and she is not sure where they have moved to.

Requests for services that the NHS does not provide seem quite normal to many of our ethnic patients but set up a lot of tension for the doctor who knows that she cannot provide them. A patient from the Asian subcontinent asks me for a 'Med 3' – a sick note for three months so that he can go and visit his estates 'back home'. He has seven workers there and they need supervision and instruction. Farzana, from the same area, asks me to prescribe medicines for a family member. "But it is so expensive back home and the medicine here is so much better," she says.

I explain to the owner of the estate that sick notes are issued according to carefully defined rules and his request is not included within them. I explain to Farzana that the NHS cannot provide medicines for people abroad – and she is asking me to prescribe treatment for someone I have never met, much less examined or assessed. Farzana is genuinely confused. "But Dr Rafiq does that all the time! Why can't you?" When Zofi asks for her sister's medicine back in her home country, she is doing something that in her culture is entirely normal.

A young Yemeni man comes to ask for rehousing. Like many people, he believes that family doctors have moles in the Housing Department. His wife is lonely because the family live in an all-white area and they would like to live with Yemenis.

A mine field opens in front of us. I do not have the power to say that rehousing is necessary on health grounds, and I certainly have no warrant to ask for rehousing on grounds of ethnicity even if I thought it proper. My Yemeni friend is genuinely confused.

Why? He thinks that I have power that I do not have, but he also feels that, as his doctor, I am his advocate and a resource. Should I not be on his side, right or wrong?

These inappropriate requests cause stress to the doctor because we just don't like saying 'no' and people don't like hearing it. But it does help to realise that these requests come out of a home culture where such requests are legitimate. Moreover, as we have seen and we will discuss again later, saying 'no' leads to a complete lack of comprehension in some cultures, Yemeni included, where playing to certain cultural rules means the answer will be 'yes'.

- **Private Medicine**

Most family doctors and nurses in Britain have very little experience of private medicine, but in many countries where incomers are from it is the mainstay of health care. It is not really a system at all but a laissez-faire business that exists for the benefit of doctors and the firms that support them. As such, patients develop skills that enable them to make use of the service.

A crucial difference is very likely to be the absence of a primary care system. This first port of call, which in UK deals with about 90% of all health care needs, does not exist or hardly exists in the home countries of most of our ethnic communities. The nearest equivalent might be in government clinics and too often this is a bad experience. Waiting times may be long and the clinics themselves dirty and unhygienic.

A newly graduated doctor in Jordan hardly draws breath before she embarks on specialist training. She has no opportunity to become a rounded general physician before specializing.

With no 'gate keeper' the patient is forced to choose a speciality to suit their problem. This, as often as not, relies on relationships and can frequently be inappropriate, causing much wasted expense and time.

It also leads to an attitude among people generally that the GP is the lowest form of medical life. If you are a British GP, and your ethnic patients assume that your specialist consultant colleagues are superior to you in both rank and expertise, you may feel your hackles rising. Calm down! This is where it comes from. Your patients will gradually become aware that you are as well qualified and as specialized in your own field as your hospital colleagues.

A friend, the pastor of a church in the Middle East, felt unwell on Friday night. He rang his urologist friend. Within two hours he was in a private hospital. Over the next two days, he endured several invasive, expensive and unpleasant procedures. On Monday, I saw him in the refugee clinic where I was working. He had been discharged and was nearly better but felt he should have a check-up 'just in case'. He was relieved that this was a wonderful opportunity to do nothing.

My pastor friend in no way doubted that that the procedures he had so stoically endured were necessary; in fact, he expected them, and I am sure his doctors did not doubt it either. The patient's expectations are that all of modern medicine and its technology will be deployed and doctors know that if this is not all done, and seen to be done, the patient and his family is likely to consider them negligent or inefficient. What if he dies? Why did the doctor not carry out every conceivable investigation and procedure? The family of the patient may well come and beat up the doctor to within an inch of his life. It is money, but not just the money. It is expectations and the culture. Where money fuels the system, why not offer more money and get better service?

Someone coming to the UK from the Middle East, or anywhere in the Asian subcontinent where this culture prevails, will be bringing the same expectations and accessing skills with them. When there is no money at stake, it removes a brake on demand, which is problematical for those of us born in this country and is much more confusing for recent arrivals. 'Free at the time of delivery' presumably means just that – free. Perhaps 'Paid for by the time of delivery' would be a more appropriate slogan.

In countries where such private medicine prevails, the government health service is likely to be at the very bottom of the pile. I have seen a group of security men putting their shoulders to the gates of a Khartoum hospital against a crowd of desperate patients. I have seen arrogant young doctors treating old ladies rudely and shamefully. I have worked in government hospitals where the toilets were so disgusting that I have been driven to scrub them myself. If some of your patients seem to be behaving unreasonably, it may be that they are coming out of this kind of experience. However good the service is in the NHS, and it is *very* good nearly all the time, your ethnic patients will often be tempted to suggest private care in the belief that it will be better.

Part 3 –More Customs and Barriers.

- **The Veil**

In the Gulf States in the 1960s (the 'Trucial Oman', as it was then called), not a single Arab woman left home without a '*burka*', a beak-like structure made of stiff material that covered all of her face, except for two slits that revealed the eyes, perhaps darkly and attractively outlined with kohl. The *burka* was almost invariably black, and the lady wore black over her head and down to her feet. I sagely prophesied that in a few years all this would have disappeared and ladies would go about with their faces open to the world.

Just how wrong can you be? In the intervening years, there has been a revival of the veil and all its varied forms. The *burka* is as entrenched as ever.

Some years later, I was living in a flat in Port Sudan on the Red Sea. On the ground floor was a doctor's surgery; the dusty street outside was part doctor's waiting room, part taxi rank and bus stop, part stopping place for goats and camels. The ladies of the Rashaida tribe would sit in a row against the wall and, adroitly flipping out a breast, would feed their babies. Their highly embroidered veils were tucked under their noses with eyes clearly visible.

A few years later, I could not help noticing the modesty and grace of the women medical students in the university. They nearly all covered their hair with a scarf that framed their faces, leaving face and eyes fully visible. They wore clothes that did not expose their bodies. There was (for the most part) an absence of courtship display, though skin tight jeans were far from rare. A very few girls wore the full *niqab*, with face and eyes completely covered. In a communications course this presented some difficulty and was not without irony.

I felt that this was very much a 'woman thing'. I went to see Dr Amina, the Iraqi lecturer in public health.

"Don't talk to me about this!" she exclaimed. "It's such a problem; it makes the rest of us feel we are inferior Muslims. Is that what they want us to feel? I've spoken to some of the girls and it makes no difference; they don't seem to understand the difficulty most of us have with *niqab*, and they have absolutely no insight as to how it will affect their patients!"

This sentiment has been echoed by other Muslim women I have known. "Are they trying make me feel I am not a good Muslim? It gives me the creeps!" said a Sheffield practice manager.

If the veil is a problem within Islam then it is not likely to be easier for the rest of us.

A Muslim lady will not wear the veil at home when she is among women, and in the presence of close male relatives, such as her brothers and her husband. The full veil or *niqab*, in which the entire face and eyes are covered (and maybe the hands as well) is essentially for the public arena. Theoretically worn so that she is protected from the prying and lecherous eyes of men, it is in fact a symbol of prosperity and status as much as anything else. In the subcontinent, the peasant life where women work as hard as men – or harder – is not conducive to the veil. When a man makes a bit of money, he can afford for his wife not to work and to impose a degree of seclusion that the veil implies. The veil then becomes a symbol of increased social status. Additionally, it is hardly necessary to point out that there is great variety in the form that the veil takes. The veil is as much an indicator of the wearer's people, family, individual family customs and branch of Islam as much as of Islam per se. To wear the veil as a sign of individual devotion is a Western gloss, as are all the political overtones.

A lady doctor is not likely to have too much of a problem if there are no men around; a man doctor more so, though I have to say that problems nearly always evaporate in the consulting room. Most women patients I have known have just thrown back their veil, to reveal a perfectly normal girl or woman wearing normal or even outrageous clothes. One young woman was wearing a full length furry imitation leopard skin leotard, another a Manchester United football shirt. The unsmiling and threatening look of the full veil has a laughing and smiling girl or woman beneath. We get on with the consultation.

A lady once attended for a sore throat. We had already met a couple of times.

"How about you lifting your veil?" I said. "After all, we do know each other pretty well now!"

"I'd prefer not, if you don't mind," she said.

"Ok then..." I gave in. "So, what's the problem?"

"I've got a sore throat."

"Well, we're not going to get very far if I can't have a look!" I said. She laughed and threw back her veil and exposed a couple of swollen and red tonsils.

Very rarely a lady announces that she is just not going to remove her veil. The wife of a Libyan gentleman never unveiled. Here was a problem because she was not the patient. She backed up her husband, a very quiet man suffering deeply from post-traumatic stress disorder, and she would berate me for failing to arrange for the family to be rehoused.

So a veiled lady comes through the door, and you are a male doctor. First, as she comes in, a gust of politics, sociology, prejudice, ignorance and perhaps tension blows in with her. You have no idea what is behind the black veil and she does not know what she is doing to you. All this needs to be acknowledged and dispelled, at least in your own mind.

Second, there may be mistrust, and some hypocrisy. The impression of sincere religious piety may not be true. Many years ago, while I was getting onto a bus, the lady next to me ran her hand up my arm inside my shirt and onto my chest. A few days later the same thing happened in the street. That was when I gave up wearing short sleeved shirts. Both women were wearing the full veil. This happened in Sudan, where there is a healthy joke culture, and where the wearing of *niqab* is taken with a large pinch of salt.

As time goes on and you get to know the ladies who are veiled, you will learn to recognise them with other cues. A brief explanation of the disadvantages that the veil brings is likely to help and she might not have appreciated these. After all, *she* can see *you*. She can also hear you, but her veil is likely to muffle her voice, causing additional difficulties. However, most times, as above, the lady quickly throws back her veil, revealing a perfectly normal person underneath and the spell is broken.

Women cannot be expected to have considered the importance of communication in the consultation– or in any area of medical or nursing practice, in hospital or in the community. However, we now accept that communication is part and parcel of clinical care and definitely *not* an optional extra. If you can't communicate well, you can't do medicine or clinical care up to the standard that we require in this country. Furthermore, the head and face, as well as the hands, give many clues as to the presence of disease or health, both mental and physical. If we cannot see the face, we can miss a world of information and it is hard or impossible to develop rapport.

If a lady was uncomfortable to the extent that she needed to remain veiled, I would suggest that she arrange to see a lady doctor. With standards as they are today, a proper consultation cannot take place with a patient fully veiled.

It is rather more difficult when the lady is not the patient and yet is still part of the consultation, as was the Libyan lady I mentioned above. An Arab lady cordially decided that she would prefer to see a lady doctor but still brought her children to see me. She remained veiled during these consultations and it was clear that the children themselves were unused to this and found the way that their mother dressed a little confusing. They would try to get behind her veil and she would try vainly to keep it in place. Eventually, we agreed that the children came with a male member of the family. Both children and doctor were happy. Later, we appointed a female colleague and the problem solved itself. But in the case of the Libyan gentleman, much later and in another practice where there was no lady doctor, we never came to any agreement.

Where the tension is likely to ratchet up is when male honour is involved. In some cultures, the honour of the family and the men is closely bound up with the seclusion of women and what they wear. This explains why in many communities the men will be seen wearing western dress but most of the women will be wearing the clothing of their 'home' country.

When a woman who is normally veiled is seen unveiled by a man who is not a close male relative or friend, honour may be violated and deep offence caused, stress and confusion reign and the consultation starts to unravel. The only time I have ever had problems in this area is if a husband or male relative comes to a consultation where a veiled woman is the patient. Left to themselves women are almost invariably fine with lifting their veil. The presence of a man alters the situation radically and the woman may not be able to say anything that conflicts with the man's point of view.

The consultation, or any medical encounter, is absolutely not the place for these tensions to be played out and I would strongly suggest that we adopt the principle that clinical care cannot be given to the standards required when the patient, or their most significant carer, is veiled. In cases where distress or offence may be caused, we (or they) need to make arrangements for the patient to be seen in a situation where they feel free to unveil in a happy and relaxed manner and not under pressure.

When it comes to health care professionals, it would seem most inappropriate that a doctor or a nurse see patients when they themselves are fully veiled. GMC guidelines do not expressly address this matter, and it is likely that patients will be inhibited from requesting to see an unveiled doctor for fear of being labelled racist. It would be good if the GMC addressed this before a cause celebre arises and finds them unprepared.

One would hope that discerning and reflective Muslims will ponder the effect of *niqab* on people who are not Muslims, when the wearer and those with them may not be fully aware of the effect that it can have, and which is probably entirely unintended.

- **The Handshake**

Your next patient walks through the door – and keeps her hands firmly to her sides as you offer her a handshake. It is a dreadful start to the consultation. If you, as a man, extend your hand to a lady from another culture and she does not reciprocate, she may not realise that to refuse a handshake in Britain is a calculated insult… and very rare.

A lady from Somalia was standing in for our regular interpreter. I wanted her to feel welcome and at home and extended my hand. When she declined to shake hands I was (inwardly) furious and deeply offended. Later, I was able to take her on one side when she explained that this was her normal habit. She was dimly aware that there was a problem but had no idea now insulting it was. She was mortified. No one had explained to her. How very British!

In Jordan, many women do not shake hands, but when a man extends his hand she will place her own right hand over her upper chest and incline her head forward ever so slightly. This serves as an indication that the lady does not shake hands and is accepted as the equivalent; everyone is happy. But we do not have the same gesture in Britain. It is possible that in time one will evolve. In my own practice, men did not offer to shake hands with women from the Asian subcontinent so the problem was resolved that way.

There are Jewish and Islamic groupings where men do not shake hands with women; if this is the case, a lady doctor might well find herself in the same situation. Here is an example of religious and/or cultural practice of one culture colliding with common politeness of another with a risk of very serious offence being taken.

- **Body Language**

"You don't like us."

I was dumbfounded and confused. I thought that we were getting on rather well.

My Korean friend repeated himself. I was mystified and explained that there was no feeling of animosity whatsoever. In fact, we were rather relishing getting to know one another.

"But you stand so far away from us!" he explained.

As we explored this further, a cultural pitfall was revealed. Koreans, it appeared, stand quite close together when they talk. The British, on the other hand, prefer a little bit of distance. Our ideas of face to face 'personal space' were slightly different. More importantly, this very difference had a significance in the politeness of Korean culture that was entirely lost on us British. We worked this one out and, with a little bit of laughter and understanding, the problem was solved.

There is a gesture in the Middle East that is essential to life. The right hand is held out, palm upwards, with the tips of the fingers and thumb together. When I do this I am saying, 'Wait a moment. Let me get a word in. Please let me into the traffic…' and some other things too. But, in some cultures, it is an obscene gesture. My friends warn me against using it in Italy, but in Jordan life comes to a standstill without it.

When I arrived in the Gulf States as a young army officer, I had the amazing privilege of working among Bedouin Arabs. On my first day, a lovely old sheikh welcomed me into his tent, and gently grasping my hand, led me into his home. I cringed inwardly, unprepared for this welcoming gesture, my mind bursting with all the baggage of my British culture. He did not let me go for some minutes. Over the next few weeks, I discovered that this was entirely normal. Men held hands frequently. But men and women? Never! Holding hands was a social gesture entirely lacking any sexual content.

So you thought with body language you were safe? Think again! We are all aware of how body language communicates our attention or lack of it, our concern or indifference. The trouble is, body signals, with dress and social gestures, can be even more confusing than words. The Somali lady had no idea that her withholding a handshake could cause deep offence. The family in Port Sudan failed entirely to understand that in doing a careful examination of their baby I was communicating that I was exercising proper care. The lady in full veil has little idea that this communicates a message that she most likely does not want to transmit. And we are hardly aware that as we touch a patient or relative the message they receive may not be at all the one we think we are sending. All cultures have strict and subtle rules about who may touch whom. Break these rules and misunderstanding and perhaps offence is the result. Fortunately, laughter and tolerance are not entirely absent on either side. Explanation and apologies go along way as long as things are brought out into the open.

- **Nursing**

Doctors enjoy high social status in most parts of the world. Sadly, the same cannot be said for nurses. Caring for the sick has been part of the Judeo-Christian culture in Britain. There is also a lot of history, and a certain amount of romance, exemplified by Florence nightingale, Edith Cavell and other famous and heroic nurses. This is built on a long tradition of monks and nuns caring for the sick. As a result, nurses are highly respected and valued; both their professionalism and vocation are equally recognised.

The same cannot be said for many of the countries that are home to immigrants to the UK. In some cultures it is shameful for women to touch men as they care for them, as nurses are bound to do. It was observable in hospitals in Birmingham three decades ago that the number of nurses whose home countries were in the Middle East or the Asian subcontinent was far lower than the number of doctors from the same countries.

So marked was this that when I encountered a nurse who was obviously from Pakistan I asked her if I could perhaps ask her a few questions about her motivation and calling. Her reply I quote verbatim. "I do this as my personal statement of rebellion against my culture."

Further afield, the president of the Faculty of Nursing at Bethlehem University in the West Bank tells me that her lifetime professional aim is to raise the status of nursing and respect for nurses from its present miserable level.

In the Middle East a hospital admission, even in a very expensive private hospital, is to experience very mediocre nursing. Perhaps, if you are fortunate to be ill enough or rich enough to be admitted to ITU, the nursing will be adequate. In many parts of Africa, the relatives of a patient in hospital are expected to undertake a good deal of the care that hospital staff do in the UK, such as washing and feeding. The nurses put up drips, give injections and other treatment but do not 'care' for the patient at all.

I stress that there are many vary honourable exceptions. In South Sudan I was deeply impressed by many of the nurses. Salaries were routinely months late and often nursing staff worked for long periods with no (official) wages.

A midwife remarked that she had not seen any salary for three months. Why did she continue?

"I'm a midwife," she answered. "That's what I do."

It said everything. Nevertheless, I do not fear to generalise.

Why am I saying all this? Because patients from countries where nursing is looked down on, training scanty and supervision inadequate may bring their suspicions, or even contempt, of nursing to this country. This may give rise to deep offence to nurses who are diligent and professional. If you are a nurse, you may be privately outraged at the way you are treated. This is where it comes from.

- **Shame**

Half a century or so ago, a woman who fell pregnant out of wedlock could be put out of her home into the street. We recoil in horror at such treatment, but why did it happen?

The culture of shame and honour has virtually disappeared from Britain, so such an act like this seems incomprehensibly cruel. Our culture has forgotten the immense power of shame. Divorce, elopement and adultery were unmentionable. Homosexuality was beyond the pale. A cleft lip was the most terrible misfortune. There was a social stigma attached to tuberculosis. There is still some shame around mental illness, but the deep disgrace that was experienced a century or so ago has all but vanished. This is wholly a good thing because shame has nothing to do with guilt or wrong doing, it is to do with public standing, reputation and 'respectability'. For a native-born British person whose family has been in this country for centuries, it is next to impossible to understand or empathise with, for instance, a man of Pakistani heritage who finds his daughter is about to marry a man who has not been chosen by him. (Or, in fact, by his wife, who is the one who has physical access to the eligible women in another family.) This choice might have been made when the children were infants and the father feels deeply shamed that his daughter is, as he sees it, in public rebellion against him.

We might be shocked when we read about honour killings, but these arise out of the deep shame experienced corporately by the family that sees a girl (and it is nearly always a girl) who marries or elopes with a man who is not the father's choice or the agreed and settled choice of the family at large.

This shame does not exist in a vacuum. It arises out of a different idea of marriage, the different status of women, and the fact that the honour of men and family is deeply invested in the 'proper' behaviour of 'their' women. The father's honour is also dependent on the need to have male children to assert his status. In some countries in the Middle East, a man ceases to be called by his name on the birth of a son, when he will be called 'Abu' before the son's name. Examples are 'Abu Ahmed' or 'Abu Mohammed' if a man has no male children he cannot, to his shame, be called Abu anything.

The culture of honour and shame runs very deep. You will encounter this in your cross-cultural practice, but where the fault lines precisely lie is for you to find out. They are different in every cultural grouping. What is clear is that shame and honour impinge on the way health matters are seen. Among the nomads of northern Sudan, the shame attached to suffering from tuberculosis was so great that patients invariably presented late when they were already very ill. Occasionally and tragically, they did not present at all, with fatal consequences.

So what? Is TB really that important? Well, it is. TB is persistently under diagnosed and has a lower index of suspicion than it deserves. It's more common among immigrants from countries where the standard of living and health is lower than our own, and is the inevitable consequence of war, displacement, malnutrition and overcrowding. The rise in TB cases seen in the refugee camps of northern Jordan and southern Syria are the direct result of the civil war. And these are countries where the shame and fear attached to TB are most marked. Compounding this is the reluctance of health care professionals to treat patients with TB, though this has lessened in recent years. Our own country has a rigorous screening programme but is far from fool proof. There are going to be cases of TB and they may well be concealed by the unfortunate sufferers because of the perceived shame that they will bring upon themselves and their families.

Far more common than TB is mental illness. In many cultures, mental illness is seen as shameful and immigrants will bring this shame with them. Frequently, mental illness is 'somatised' and becomes a physical problem, with all the language of physical illness that comes with it. 'Total body pain', and all the syndromes that are linked with it, all the frustrating symptoms that have required multiple and fruitless investigation, have their roots here.

Another area linked to shame is mental and physical disability, especially congenital. In many cultures, a disabled child will be kept at home out of sight, and away from the gaze of neighbours. They may well feel that God is visiting them with judgment or that they have been cursed – of which more below.

A further deep cause of shame is infertility, with the family disgrace compounding the personal pain. And so often it is assumed that the lady is to blame: it is 'her fault'. Even the perceived inability to produce a son can be a cause of shame, again with the woman taking the 'blame'. When a couple (or far more likely, the woman) talks to you about her inability to conceive, the idea of combined cause and the possibility that her husband may have something to do with it needs to be tactfully suggested. Initially, a husband might react strongly to the suggestion, but the assurance that the whole matter will be treated with the utmost confidentiality usually helps him to come round.

But the honour and shame culture is not restricted to the Middle East and the subcontinent. Zofi's husband clearly expects to dictate the outcome of the encounter with Dr Rosina. The fact that he does not get his way may well be the cause of shame or 'loss of face'. This is not a power encounter, in that he is not using the event to demonstrate his authority: it is just that, as husband and father, this is the way things are at home and he does not stop to think that this is not how things work here. But he may 'lose face' and take it out on his wife, whose perceived weakness may be the cause of his embarrassment.

Shame and honour can suddenly invade the ward or the consulting room. Virtually all men born in Britain accept that rectal examinations are a necessary if unpleasant part of being over forty-five years old.

Your Asian or Arab patients may not be so compliant and may quite possibly be outraged at the suggestion. The 'rules' governing examinations may be equally difficult for the unwary.

In far Eastern cultures, suffering and disability can be held to be due to 'Bad Karma' – if you have led a bad life in your former incarnation then it is possible that you will suffer trauma in this one. A disabled child is very possibly someone who has been wicked in a former life – or perhaps it is you yourself who are being punished. This removes the need for compassion and kindness to the sufferer. Why should I be kind or try to alleviate the suffering of one who richly deserves it?

- **Magic and the Occult**

Fatima is every inch a Brummie girl, born and bred, and in her third year reading electronics at university. She is telling me about her mother-in-law. A few years ago a surgical operation went tragically wrong and she is now in a wheelchair. Lawyers decided that the surgical team was to blame and the NHS parted with a substantial sum in consequence.

But that is not at all how Fatima sees it. "They got it all wrong, Doc," she says. Actually, we paid a *pir* (an imam, recognised to have out of the ordinary spiritual powers) to fast for forty days. At the end of that, he said that we should send home to Pakistan and get someone to dig down to the foundations of our house, and there we would find her name written on one of the stones. We did, and there it was, just like he said, together with a curse written there. That's why she's like she is."

Fatima is an educated British girl but her world view is entirely different from that of her native English contemporaries. If it is hard for us, as a virtually shame-free culture, to understand the profound effects of honour and shame, it is even harder for a secularist with a materialist world view to understand the world as perceived by most of our Asian and Middle Eastern friends.

Fatima and her family live in a world that is peopled with spiritual beings: djinns, evil and not so evil; angels, good and bad; and people who, like the *pir* above, have spiritual power, whether good or not so good. There is *Baraka* (blessing, or some other benefit such as financial, or in particular, healing) to be sought for, or misfortune or evil to be warded off, often in the form of the evil eye that can cause harm, especially to children or pregnant women. There are special people around who have the ability to transmit *Baraka* in one way or another, and there are other people who can curse and cause harm.

I am on a home visit. There is a scrap of paper rather bizarrely taped to the window pane. "It's the neighbours," says Salima Begum. "They give us the eye. She's always looking over here. The *pir* gave me this, and told me to stick it on the window where she looks in." She takes it down and shows it to me; it is a hand written verse from the Qur'an. She replaces it carefully on the window pane.

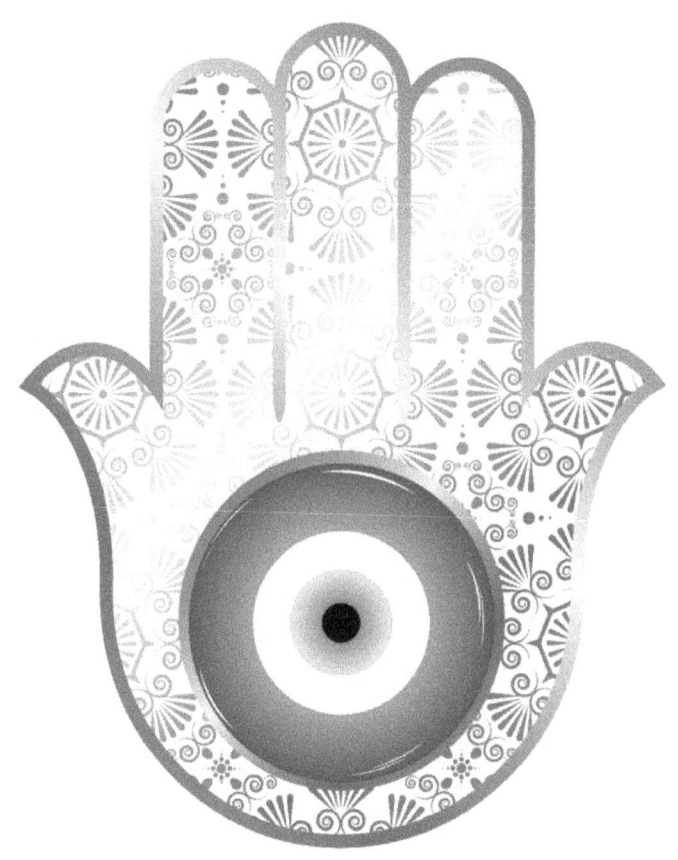

Protection against the 'evil eye'

The evil eye belief extends far beyond the subcontinent; it is widespread in rural and not so rural communities all across North Africa, South America and southern Europe, as well as Celtic communities in the British Isles. It is immensely ancient and there is evidence of its presence in Mesopotamia more than five thousand years ago. And it is deeply influential in how people see the causation of disease and misfortune.

Much of this is bound up with healing, health and disease, but also in negotiating the vagaries of modern life. Two teenage girls are wearing *taweez* (amulets) round their necks and I ask what they are for. "It's for my GCSE's," says the first. "I'm not sure I've really done the work, but I really need good grades." And what about your sister? "Oh, I like to watch horror movies," she says; "I wear *taweez* so afterwards I don't get bad dreams." I ask where they obtained these *taweez,* tiny boxes on black thread that they are wearing round their necks. "Our nan gave them us when we were back home in the summer," comes the reply.

Among Muslim families these little amulets are tiny boxes that contain a piece of paper on which is written a verse of the Qur'an and are placed round the neck of an adult or a child. There are countless other kinds common in other cultures.

Rabia brings her little boy to the surgery. "He's got the runs something terrible," she tells me.

Rabia's little boy has an amulet round his neck. "So, where does this come from?" I ask.

"Oh… My mum gave it to me. She said it would make him better."

"Has it worked?"

Rabia laughs. "Not a lot!"

Rabia, like everyone else I know, has not the slightest difficulty in seamlessly integrating magic with modern medicine. She uses both.

Occult and magic practices occur with bewildering variety, with every family following different variations. I have heard dozens of remedies against the evil eye, from the one above, using talismans and Qur'anic verses, to mixing a variety of herbs and then eating or setting fire to the resulting mixture, to watching the ground where a person suspected of having the 'evil eye' has walked and then hammering a nail into the floor where her (and it is nearly always 'her') foot has trodden.

Generally, magic is in the hands of women, particularly in the case of the evil eye, but most of the time men go along with it 'just in case.' However, the subject is far from esoteric. If you ask about it, people will talk! But there are ways of asking that we will talk about in the third section.

- **Qat**

In the middle of the crossroads the traffic policeman stands with his bootlaces around his ankles. The Sana'a traffic hurtles round him, ignoring his attempts to direct it. He has what looks like a cricket ball tucked into his left cheek. The bulge is his afternoon chew of *qat*. No wonder the Arabic word for chewing *qat* is 'to store'. Mostly done in groups, the afternoon is often taken up with chewing *qat* in the company of one's male friends. The leaves are lovingly stroked, then taken into the mouth. They are not swallowed, but disgorged in a deluge of green slime all at once at the end of the session. Women do chew as well but, like most other activities in Yemen, men and women *qat* chewing parties are segregated.

No doubt my policeman is probably retired now and, in all likelihood, some of his children and grandchildren are living in Balsall Heath, (Birmingham) or Firvale (Sheffield). They are likely to be chewing *qat*, though not on such a large scale, and unlike their grandfather, the policeman. they will not be as skinny and undernourished as a result,

The effects of *qat* are subtle:[ii] "Optimism, mild euphoria, excitation, talkativeness, increased energy, and enhanced self-esteem. The half-life is about four hours, depending on the amount of chewed khat (sic). When the acute effects vanish, users experience feelings of depletion, insomnia, numbness." However, most people suffer few ill effects. Your taxi driver in Yemen will not drive as though drunk, but he will drive too fast for comfort. A drive through the mountains in a service taxi had me in the ditching position on many occasions as we missed the dizzy precipitous ravines by inches. The 'high' is subtly different from the high of cannabis, and people are able to function to a degree. But, if you are in Yemen, don't go to a government office after midday; you will achieve nothing. And don't visit your friend's house unless you are prepared to join in the 'chew'.

Qat is not physically addictive, but there is a powerful social habit that reinforces its use. However, the use of *qat* in the UK is a standing argument for the legalisation of drugs. *Qat* is entirely legal and there is no criminal activity associated with it.

Qat will only grow above about 5,000 feet, so mercifully the habit is really restricted to the mountainous countries of the Middle East and East Africa, i.e. Yemen and the horn of Africa.

It is surprising how little the observable effects are in view of the drug's regular and continual use by so many. But where there are psychiatric problems and gastrointestinal issues, it is worth bearing the habit in mind if your patient or their family is from a *qat* chewing region, i.e. Somalia, Ethiopia Eritrea or Yemen.

- **FGM and Other Cultural Issues.**[iii]

"I will never marry a woman who has been cut," said the young nomad. "I will need to marry a foreigner!"

"I will never, *never* allow my little girls to be cut." This from the father of three girls. "All the women in our family have had it, but it stops here."

The Nomads of Eastern Sudan practice the most extreme form of FGM, or clitoridectomy as it is sometimes called. It is also in practical terms universal in that culture. This is an entirely female project, carried out by women and reinforced by the older ladies. It taps into deeply held beliefs about female purity and cleanliness. To not have it done renders a woman unclean and 'unpurifed'. It is also a virtually indispensable rite of passage rendering a girl adult and ready for marriage.

There are also notions about the taming of the ungovernable sexual desire of women and making women more attractive to men but, whenever the subject came up among men (and it came up rather frequently, suggesting a level of concern), there was almost universal disapproval and dislike of the practice, as the remarks above suggest. There seems to be a disconnect between what men think and feel and what women believe. In a society where there are such high social barriers between men and women, this is hardly surprising. One sex is doing it for the supposed benefit on the other. Many (perhaps most) of the 'other' do not agree with it at all.

Somali people practice a similar form of FGM and this is also universal in the culture; the beliefs that it represents, and its practice are prevalent in Somali communities in UK in spite of its illegal status. My experience in Sudan confirms my impression that this practice is deeply abusive and traumatic to the women who have it inflicted on them, often leading to a degree of mental illness, quite apart from physical problems; difficulty urinating, and many urinary tract infections being one. Ironically, its effect on sexual satisfaction and desire is certainly not proven.

Visually, FGM is shocking. The normal contours of the vulva are obliterated and replaced by dry, hard and unyielding scar tissue.

Any doctor or nurse, midwife or health visitor will want to build up a picture of its prevalence. Of course, women practitioners will be at an advantage, and midwives a greater advantage still, but male workers have their part to play. In view of the remarks that I have quoted, it is worth men having 'man to man' talks with male family members. You can slowly build up a picture of how prevalent FGM is and what people feel about it. It is possible that men might hold the key to eradicating the practice of FGM.

But FGM is not an isolated issue: it comes with other features of cultures that have lately arrived in Britain and underlines the deep gulf that exists between our different cultures and values. We are treading on dangerous ground when we start to judge the culture and habits of others, yet we cannot practice our profession in a moral, legal or ethical vacuum.

I said right at the beginning that we need to have a critical view of our own cultures before we judge anyone else's. We cannot judge other cultures simply by using our own as a criteria. But it hardly needs saying that FGM, slavery, people trafficking and gender-based abortion are all illegal, and they is also *wrong.* That is a moral judgment that our society makes. These judgments are in turn based on the Christian ethic that underlines so much of our medical culture, and which I for one share. To make sense of these values, practitioners from other cultures and religions will without doubt find their own ideological foundation. Medical people, especially midwives, district nurses and others working in the community will be well placed to identify FGM as well as abortion on the grounds of gender, and perhaps slavery and people trafficking.

You will doubtless be thinking this over bearing in mind the ethics of the British medical profession. So many cultural features that I have mentioned are to do with the poor and the marginalised. As health people in the state health service we have a responsibility to look out for them.

- **Gender**

Ahmed lives in Balsall Heath, Birmingham, but his father, Abu Ahmed, was a farmer in Yemen until he came to the UK. Abu Ahmed has been having trouble with his water works. Finally, his family persuades the old man to attend his GP. In desperation, he goes, not thinking very deeply about who will see him or what they will do.

Imagine his surprise when he finds the doctor is about the age of his son, Ahmed… worse, she is a woman! Abu Ahmed cannot talk about his waterworks to a young lady the age of his own daughter. He turns and runs for it.

Fortunately he was not around long enough to discover that part of the diagnosis involves a rectal examination, imagine his horror!

I worked in a practice in Sheffield in which every last employee, doctor and nurse were female. From the moment I was appointed, I had to become an expert in man problems. Men were queuing up to discuss their erectile dysfunction and their prostates. Was I such a great clinician or just madly popular? Neither. I was simply a bloke – and a little older.

The tolerance and relationship between male and female in the consultation is finely tuned in Britain, but your patients may come from a culture where it is equally finely tuned – but markedly different. A native English man will probably accept a rectal examination from a female doctor, but a man from a Middle Eastern culture is likely to be deeply offended at the idea of such an assault from *any* doctor, male or female, as it may well be most shameful in his own culture. In my own practice, before we appointed a lady doctor, we observed a strict protocol over examinations. All intimate female examinations were performed by our nurse practitioner, who fortunately was very experienced and professional. Examining abdomens, however, was within limits, and all our Asian patients wore the *Salwar Kamees* made of the thinnest of materials, which were easily felt through. This was found quite acceptable for me as a man, but we made sure a chaperone was invariably present.

When chaperones are necessary – and nowadays they are *always* necessary – absolutely resist the temptation to use a relative or friend. If there is any trouble the relative will end up in a very difficult position. A male colleague from Egypt was consulted by a teenage Asian girl with thrush. She asked for her sister who had come with her to be her chaperone. All went well until a few days later, when the girl's father discovered that his daughter had been examined by a male doctor. There was an incandescent family row. The father's honour was deeply wounded and the poor sister was pressured into saying that the examination had been under duress.

The situation was eventually resolved but the cost to the doctor was many months of suspension from practice and a huge amount of stress and trauma to both himself and his family. The lesson? A professional person must act as chaperone or the exam is postponed until one is available.

• Life and Death

The much-loved dean of the Jordanian medical college where I was teaching tragically suffered a most severe stroke. Three weeks after the event, he was still in intensive care, barely conscious, unable to feed himself or speak.

While I was visiting him his office manager arrived. After a moment's silence, she launched into a long speech in which she assured him at length that he was certain to recover fully. He would be back to work in a few weeks and all would undoubtedly be well.

If there is one major and deeply emotional area where we differ from Middle Eastern and African cultures it is the way we talk about life and death. The office manager was acting within her cultural bounds and this is what she *had* to say. There is a lot of collusion and hiding of the truth from each other. The dean, a doctor himself, would have known that the outcome was the opposite of what she was describing. Many others had come and said the same thing.

In our seminars, we would discuss with the medical students how to break bad news. Many would concur with the episode above. "We can't possibly tell our patients they have cancer," they would say. "They will just give up and die…"

I would explain that this is actually not usually what happens. There would be a lively debate as some of the students saw the implications of not being truthful with their patients.

One day a young medical student jumped to her feet. "We can't go on like this!" she shouted. "My auntie died two months ago – she was in dreadful pain all the time and we never told her what was going on. It was terrible; we kept telling her she was going to get better – all the dishonesty and lies… and I am sure she knew at the end…" She sat down, biting back her tears. Many of the other students were quick to agree with her.

In my own practice, I was visited by a posse of relatives representing their mother who had a clearly fatal prognosis. "You mustn't tell her doctor, you really mustn't! We want you to promise us that you won't tell her."

We negotiate carefully and eventually we come to an agreement. They agree that I will visit their home and we will ask their mother what she knows and what she wants to know, and take it from there, step by step.[iv]

- **War and Civil Disruption**

It is extraordinary how normally people can behave even when they have very recently been subjected to horrific events. The Syrian lady in the refugee clinic was chatting and laughing to her friends in the waiting area. During our encounter, I asked about her family. She disintegrated in front of my eyes. Four weeks previously her husband and four children had been killed in front of her.[v]

Those who have been subject to horrific experiences will have sustained severe emotional and psychological damage, and will suffer post-traumatic stress in varying degrees. They may outwardly appear 'normal' yet be subject to terrifying nightmares, depression or euphoria. They may have flashbacks so intense that they are catapulted back into the situation and act as if they were in it. An American friend tells me about a marine, recently returned from Afghanistan. He is in a shopping mall. He hears a loud noise and snaps instantly into combat mode, taking cover behind a car – oblivious to the people and goings on around him. It takes him a quarter of an hour to settle down and revert to the present moment. Not only does he relive the terrors of that moment but he drags his young newly married wife into his trauma and it throws huge strain on their relationship.

The sufferer is likely to experience deep anxiety, intense guilt and unbearable grief at the loss of those they love as well as possessions, home, country and their own familiar culture. On top of this, they must cope with culture shock and adaptation to a new country and home. A lady is used to sloshing water on the floor to clean her house. What does she do when confronted by a fitted carpet? She and her family may have never seen a sit-down toilet. What do they do with this, and how do they adapt their private cultural and religious customs to their new and incomprehensible environment?

Experiences of this kind should always be borne in mind – but so should the traumas of the distant past. Rafiq, a recovering heroin addict, tells me that one of his earliest memories in Pakistan is of his father killing his mother with a knife. Where cultures and families have no interior means of dealing with this, men and women are likely to suffer long term damage. Most cultures have their own methods of dealing with post-traumatic stress disorder, which are entirely different from western ways, but these corporate rituals and processes may not be readily available to those here who need them most.

Part 4 – But I'm Not British!

You have just arrived from the sub-continent or from Europe or from further afield. You are fully qualified, and you have passed the PLAB test – but the moment you walk into the street you can't understand a word that anyone is saying. Is this really English they are talking?

And they are not terribly friendly either. A little bit cold?

"I sat on the bus and everyone seemed to be in their private bubble. Even the people not looking at their phones were staring into space. And when I asked my new boss if I could call round at his house, there was a lot of mumbling and pulling out of diaries...."

- **Are We 'Cold'?**[vi]

Yes, we British are a funny lot. And the first thing you need to know about us is that we *are* a little bit cold. That is because we come from a culture where people 'keep themselves to themselves'. This is a very British phrase and sums up a lot of our social attitudes to each other. People don't do things outside; it's cold out there. We do things at home and indoors. And, even when you are at work in your hospital, your English friends don't seem to share a lot with you. It seems that life at work and life at home are kept in two different departments. Not a bit like at home.

The thing is, if you are from Africa, Pakistan or the Middle East, you come from what we might term a 'warm culture' where people live in the street and relationships matter more than getting things done. On a bus or train, you would never dream of bringing out the food that you had brought with you without offering to share it with the person next to you. In fact, all the passengers will probably end up sharing their food with each other; it's a party. Not so in Britain. We are in a bubble half the time, and public transport is a typical example. It is part of living in a cold culture. We are not very convivial publicly with strangers. I will eat my egg mayonnaise sandwich in solitary silence.

But when we get to know you, you will find us just as friendly as anyone in your own country. It will just take a little longer.

- **Relationships v. Efficiency**

Our culture emphasises efficiency – on getting things done. You might find this a bit disconcerting as it may well cut across relationships. It is possible that, in your country, relationships come before efficiency all the time. The hospital near where I worked as a primary health care doctor in Sudan functioned entirely on this principle. The Landover, whose job it was to act as an ambulance was immobilised as the driver and four assistant drivers' salaries took up the entire ambulance budget. There was no money for fuel; the vehicle was propped up on blocks and the engine provided a home for a family of mice. It was more important for the hospital staff to hire their relatives than it was for the ambulance to do its job properly.

The Relief and Development Agency that I worked with in northern Sudan worked along the same lines. If you had a friend or relative who worked for it, you might feel that your friend should get you a job in the agency, and you would be right. The office was staffed with many people whose jobs I could never really work out, but the programmes suffered because the available money was spent on extra staff. Relationships predominate; efficiency suffers.

In the same country, Kenneth, a Sudanese aid worker, would occasionally come under cover of darkness and ask, in great secrecy, if we could possibly hide for him a huge sixty-pound sack of *durra,* the country's staple grain. He would explain that, from time to time, he would come and take some of it for his wife and children and others under his roof. And would we *please* not breathe a *word* of it to a soul. The reason? He had bought this for his immediate family but, if his other relatives got wind of it, they would all be down there asking for some. And he just cannot say no to them: in that culture, you cannot say no to your relatives. Relationships are king but efficiency suffers. It is a hot culture characteristic.

In Britain and most of northern Europe we are cold cultures and we tend to value efficiency more than relationships. Your new consultant or matron is less concerned about his or her relationship with you than that you do your job well, although they will hopefully be concerned about happy relationships at work as well. Do your job well and the relationships will follow.

- **Saying 'No'**

A factor that exists in cold cultures is the ability for people to say 'no'; in direct contrast to what we have seen above. I was used to the way people say 'no' in cultures where they cannot say no to your face. I was planning a TB control programme in Sudan and had arranged an interview with a very high-flying westernised doctor who was in charge of a key national health initiative. I had been on a course that she had taught, and we had worked on the plans for a TB control project. I felt that I had a very cordial relationship with her and the interview was going to go well.

After a sixteen-hour bus ride, I arrived at her office.

"Dr Sadiqa (not her real name) isn't here. She has gone out," says her office manager with admirable tautology.

I was stunned. I had come a long way. I had an appointment.

"Will she be here in the morning?"

"Maybe. I'll tell her you called."

"Would it be alright if I saw her for a few minutes tomorrow then?"

"Perhaps… Inshallah…"

But in the morning Dr Sadiqa wasn't there. She was in a meeting.

I was getting the message. Once I get through her door and am being offered tea, the game is lost and Dr Sadiqa cannot, absolutely cannot, say no to me. So she is saying no by her absence and I need to read what is going on and not cause a lot of embarrassment by persisting. Much later, the details arrive in the form of a letter. She is indeed saying no but, even then, I have to reach the past paragraph before I get the message. Our relationship, and even my presence in her office, would have prevented here giving me the negative answer that she thought necessary.

Contrast this with an encounter I had with a Russian civil servant in Armenia. Not knowing either Russian or Armenian, I had found a very capable interpreter in Sophie, a nineteen-year-old Armenian school leaver who spoke Russian and English fluently, and had a brain to match.

I cannot remember the reason for this interview, only my shock at how it ended. We were having a very friendly chat with Sophie doing (I suppose) an excellent job as an interpreter. We had drunk sweet mint tea. We were obviously getting on well. There was laughter and some jokes that survived the language barrier. All my experience in the culture of Sudan and the Middle East told me that this was going to turn out well.

Then: "*Niet.*"

I was shocked. Had I misread the atmosphere completely? What had gone wrong?

Afterwards, Sophie just couldn't understand my confusion. "Nothing went wrong," she said. "The answer was just 'no'."

I explained where I was coming from, and my experience of the Arab world. Bewildered, she turned to me. "How can you run a country like that?" she asked in amazement.

The answer is that Armenia, and many parts of the former Soviet Union, are cold cultures. People can say 'no' and they do. Efficiency matters more than relationships. The cordiality, so carefully built up over tea and cakes, which would have achieved the desired result in one culture, was entirely irrelevant in another. And in the United Kingdom people will say 'no'. They may not be as direct as the Armenian official, they may go round the houses and be very polite, and they will wish very much that you hadn't asked in the first place, but they can, and will, say 'no'.

- **We Are Devious**

Yes, I'm afraid we are. In my culture we often don't dare complain to someone's face, so we do it behind their backs. It is a sign of social cowardice and it is an unattractive feature of life in Britain. If you are from a country where people are very direct with each other, you will be confused and shocked, and you may get into trouble because you assume people will speak up – and they don't. There may be initial embarrassment, but there is virtue in 'knowing where we are' with each other.

I was in a meeting with medical assistants and primary health care workers in South Sudan. The Chinese bicycles that we provided for them were the only ones that could withstand the battering from terrain and use and were a lifeline, an item that made their work rather less impossible, but supply lines were long and erratic.

One of them stood up. "You promised to provide me with bicycle and you have totally failed," he exclaimed.

People from such a direct and confrontational culture find our ways incomprehensible. The Somali lady who would not shake hands, who I mentioned above, had little idea of the effect she was having. She would have benefitted hugely from a little bit of brave confrontation. Be warned…

- **Racism**

Now we are entering the area of highly charged political dynamite. Are we British racist or not?

Well, it depends who you speak to, your ethnicity, how dark your skin actually is, what culture you come from, and whether you are looking for it.

A good friend, a former asylum seeker from Uganda, who now – after many years – has a decent job, finds a lot of racism. He attends a cathedral. "People accept me, but I can see that they have real difficulty," he said. He does a good deal of political advocacy for asylum seekers and finds much covert racism.

On the same day, I speak to Thomas. He is an electrician from Nigeria who has recently married an English girl and has had extensive surgery on his hips. He is finding the refugee's usual difficulty in finding a job, though he is very well qualified.

"It is great here," he says, leaning on his crutches. "I feel so at home in my church and they have been marvellous to me. Of course, you British are a very reserved lot and it takes time for you to open up. You are not like us Nigerians, who talk to each other all the time. But that's just something we have to get used to."

A Sudanese man from a nomadic people group on the Red Sea Coast is very dark skinned and is married to a Syrian lady who is white. This interracial marriage caused huge problems in Syria. "I could get in a fight any day in Damascus," he said. "Every day I got racist remarks and insults in the street. Now I live in England, I am accepted completely; that is one of the reasons I stay here."

Another Sudanese attended a three-month course at the Liverpool School of Tropical Medicine and Hygiene. On his return to Sudan, I asked him about his experiences. "The white people were fine," he laughed, "but the black people were so racist!"

As a volunteer at an asylum seeker drop-in centre, I was given a brief to look out for 'hate crime'. It became clear after a very short while that a number of asylum seekers had been subject to abuse and even violence from other asylum seekers on their way to Britain and on arrival. There was a good deal of inter-racial tension.

I was enjoying a meal at one of my favourite restaurants, a Kurdish restaurant in Burngreave, Sheffield, an area home to many language groups and immigrant communities. A fight broke out between two groups of young men. It turned out that one group were Iraqi Kurds, the other Iraqi Arabs. Later, a policeman confirmed to me that there was very little crime in that area, but a significant level of violence between ethnic groups.

I interviewed ten Chinese doctors. None had experienced any racism in the health service whatsoever. I spoke to two Eritreans at the same time who work together as domestic staff in a spinal unit. One experienced much racism and prejudice; the other said he had never experienced racism of any kind.

I suggest we can very tentatively draw out a few points.

Cultural not racial factors. Frequently, we misread cultural or political differences as racism. This may or may not be the case but we need to be aware of possible misunderstandings.

Depth of colour. Darkness of colour may be a factor in racial prejudice.

Racism is international and inter-community. It is not just white British people holding prejudice against the rest. Racism is endemic in all of us. We need to find out just how we ourselves are racist and take steps to deal with it in our own hearts.

The other point of view. Understand that people of any colour or race in the host culture have their own difficulties. We are all adapting to the huge cultural changes that are taking place all over Europe, as well as here in Britain, and we all need to give people a little slack. It is not always easy for us to get used to change.

Finally, *Harmony.* Racism gets a lot of publicity. Harmony very little. The Health Service is full of great examples of racial harmony and tolerance, but we don't hear much about them.

- **Doctor, Doctor…**

You may come from a culture where you are greatly respected as a professional and as a doctor. Doctors are well liked and respected in Britain as well, but you will find that respect is not uncritical and has to be earned. This is an excellent thing, although it has been hard for us all to get used to! None of us can be above being called to account. It is part of the post-modern perspective that authority and institutions are regarded with varying degrees of suspicion.

You might also come from an environment where you are always called 'doctor'. This will not be the case in Britain, where after a while your contemporaries and your seniors will call you by your first name. Don't be offended. We are not being rude, it is just the culture! The use of your first name will denote a degree of informality, but you had better be careful how you address your seniors, men or women. There is no harm in asking what they would like to be called, but you had better call them 'doctor' or 'matron' until they say otherwise.

- **Nurse, Nurse**

On the other hand, if you are a nurse coming into this country, you may well be surprised at the respect you receive from the general public, your patients and the doctors whom you work with. A nurse in a spinal unit said to me, "Go back to Poland? Never! I was treated like dirt there. Now I work in a team; I get to have my say in how our patients are treated, I feel respected and appreciated for my skills. No way am I ever going back!"

This has very important implications if you are a doctor. You may well have come from a culture where the nursing profession generally, and nurses in particular, are not respected and valued as they are in Britain. There is no quicker way of making enemies than treating nurses in any other way than as equal colleagues. Do not be slow to ask their advice – and to act on it too. They may well know much more than you do in their specialist field, and more about the patients under their care. They will go out of their way to help you– and keep you out of trouble as well – if they feel appreciated and respected.

- **Professional Colleagues**

While working in the Middle East, there seemed no shortage of doctors. But when a young Syrian man came to the refugee clinic with his prosthetic leg we were in trouble. Pulling up his trousers, he showed me a battered and dented piece of metal. There were extra screws everywhere and it seemed to be held together entirely by duct tape in an effort to keep it up and running. The padding in the socket was worn and ripped and covered with dried blood. Unsurprisingly, his stump was covered in agonising sores.

It was only with the utmost difficulty that we could find a technician who was able to repair this battered and worn prosthesis. As for finding a physiotherapist who could train him in the proper way to walk with it, forget it. This experience is in stark contrast with the privilege that we have in the UK. There is an army of professionals who form the back bone of the service. There are midwives and health visitors, there are physiotherapists, occupational therapists, laboratory scientists, as well as specialist technicians of every kind; then there are security men, porters, cleaners, quite apart from ward clerks, receptionists, accountants, managers and the whole leadership structure that the NHS depends on.

This army of men and women form the foundations of the NHS, which is vastly more than its doctors and nurses. If you come from a country where the doctors are used to being treated as – and behaving like – prima donnas then you are in for a shock. The health service culture works on the basis that we all treat each other with mutual respect – and that means that we respect each other's areas of expertise as well. This means asking for advice where appropriate and acting on it too. Your status as a doctor needs to be worn lightly, perhaps much more lightly than in your home country!

- **Women**

If you are a lady doctor you may well have enjoyed high status in your home country. As a nurse, as I have said before, you may well be surprised that you are treated with much greater respect in Britain, both as a woman and as a nurse. As a male doctor, you might have come from a culture where women are treated with less respect than in the UK. There is a high degree of sensitivity about male/female relationships in the public sphere and the whole area of gender relationships is highly politicised. Tread very warily, but you cannot go wrong if you treat women with great respect at all times and value their judgment and skills as on an equal level as your male colleagues.

- **Patients**

I hope that some of the remarks in earlier sections of this book will be helpful from the opposite perspective. Your patients will take your professional skills and knowledge for granted, but your facility in English, your understanding of their regional accent (of which we have many) will have a major effect on whether you will gain their confidence.

Many countries have English as the language of medicine, but the way we communicate with other members of our medical team is not the way we communicate with patients. This means that medical terms will not be appropriate and you will have to learn the street names for the words you will be more familiar with. I sometimes used to think that the severe communication problems that arose between doctors in the Middle East and their patients were made worse by the fact that doctors talked to other doctors in English and to their patients in Arabic.

Your British patients will expect you to treat them as equals in intelligence. While older members of ethnic minorities may treat you as an authority figure, their younger children and those of immigrant heritage will have a British cultural view of health staff. This means that they will regard you as accountable to them in a way that might not be the case at 'home'. In any case, do *not* expect to be treated as an authority figure! This has many practical implications. You will need to explain how you arrived at your diagnosis, and why you intend to manage things as you do. Moreover, you will need to obtain your patients' full agreement and informed consent to any treatment that you are suggesting.

- **Ethos**

As part of your induction into British medical practice, you will be introduced to British medical ethics. There may be quite difficult changes that you will need to make, and which will need much introspection by yourself, and hopefully discussion with indigenous British colleagues as well as medical staff in the same position as yourself, that is, coming from abroad. You may recognise some of the cultural factors that I have outlined earlier as being part of your own home culture. You may, for instance, come from a culture where FGM is endemic or where abortion on gender grounds is prevalent. Your adjustment to British medical practice and culture will involve the abandonment of practices that are not consistent with what is considered right here.

Part 5 – What Can We Do About It?

It is time to get back to Zofi, Dr Rosina and their disastrous encounter. Challenging as cross-cultural communication is, and the pitfalls many, there are solutions and also joys around the corner.

How can we improve things? How can we watch Zofi's back as she leaves with 'happy patient' written between her shoulder blades? How can we help Dr Rosina reach for the 'happy doctor' card in the drawer of her desk?

- **Starting Ahead Of The Game**

It was coffee time at a GP training day. A group of Asian doctors were chatting together. I saw my chance and joined them. "Tell me some secrets!" I said. "My practice is more than ninety percent Asian. How do I do it?"

Their answer surprised me. "But you have all the advantages!" one of them declared. "We are supposed to understand these people, but they are from a different social class than us professionals; they are really racist and they much prefer English doctors!"

The others agreed. Moreover, I had begun to realise that, as a doctor entirely out of the culture of my clientele, I had some major advantages. There seemed to be huge respect for the health service and its ethos, even when unrealistic expectations were voiced. We have looked at the dubious practices and even corruption that is a feature of many health services worldwide; my patients from the subcontinent seemed to think that the NHS was fairly incorruptible. They are not too far wrong. Here are some other factors that are working on our side.

- **Confidentiality**

Our patients valued our ethos of confidentiality very highly. The 'shared privacy' of many Asian homes was anathema to the younger generation who wanted what they talked about to stay within the four walls of the consulting room. Many teenagers would so have liked to have had better access to their school teachers, but this did not seem possible except on a very occasional basis. But their GP? Well, they could just go in there and the door would shut behind them – and they could talk. And talk they did. And not only teenagers; when older people, first generation immigrants from the subcontinent, realised that there was absolute confidentiality, they came in their droves. Once the men had decided that I was harmless, women started to come on their own. They welcomed the chance to talk without their husbands and, perhaps more importantly, behaved 'normally' and not in the assumed cultural way that women were expected to behave when their husbands or other male family members were present.

I used to ask new patients why they had changed practices and why they had chosen this one when there were doctors from their own country and culture on every street corner. Confidentiality was invariably the first answer they gave. "If I go to my mum's doctor, she'll know every word I said before I get home!" said Parveen.

"We know *you* won't tell anyone what we are talking about because you're not in our culture," a young man said to me. Being outside the culture, along with confidentiality, was almost invariably the reason people gave for coming to the practice.

- **Accessibility**

NHS staff, especially general practitioners and their own staff, are seen to be available all the time. In my own practice, there was no appointment system, an arrangement that suited the local culture. My various attempts to introduce an appointment system were met with universal horror. People explained that they came to meet their friends and that often a visit to the surgery was a social occasion thinly veiled as a medical visit. In a culture with a fairly high degree of seclusion, one of the places a woman could freely go to was the surgery. And go they did.

What was our response? We could make the surgery doctor friendly or patient friendly. We decided on the latter even though it was far harder work, and cost more too. But it was much more satisfying and much more fun.

And often the harder work was brought on by the fact that a lady – or her husband – would bring all the children to the surgery. Our receptionist would remonstrate. "Do you really want all the children to be seen?" "Yes!" would be the answer.

Once a community from another culture reaches a critical size, it becomes hard for any member of it to make contact with individuals outside. This is problematic for younger people, especially those who are second generation incomers who are growing up to be British Asians or Africans and are, at the same time, being heavily imbued with their parent's culture. Many are trying to get away from their background and feel imprisoned within it. Parents, for their part, are often disarmingly frank about their desire to inculcate the values of their own cultures into their children in an attempt to make them grow up like children in their country of origin. They are often confused as they see that somehow this is not happening.

- **Education**

Education is so different from 'home' that first generation parents have very little idea what is going on in a British school and wonder why their children are turning out so different from themselves.

The evening English-as-a-second-language class is in full swing. The teacher says a word. The students repeat it. On and on it goes, sing song and, it seems, a bit mindless. We are in Port Sudan and the class is made up of Arabs, Nomads and African people from South Sudan. Here people are educated by rote. The teacher has a very high social status and his word is not to be questioned. In the Middle East and Africa, I have had my use of English criticised. Why? Am I not a native English speaker? No! This is what our teacher says and he is right![vii]

When refugees or migrants arrive in this country, they find that this kind of teaching English is less than ideal and they can't understand a word of English. They then have the opportunity to go to a class where the teachers are trained differently and the courses enable them to obtain a reasonable grasp of the language.

Education in some parts of the subcontinent is heavily didactic and is built round the idea that there is a body of knowledge to be communicated and taken on board. My visit to two mosque schools exemplified this; the teacher was reading the words copied on the blackboard. The students were repeating them and learning them by heart. There was not too much explanation and no dialogue with the students.

In contrast, education in this country will give children, especially girls, a sense of their own identity rather than of their role, and also open their eyes to a huge range of opportunities in life. It is little wonder that parents are sometimes confused as to the way their children were turning out. Many young girl patients loved school and viewed with alarm the prospect of attending a school built round their own culture and religion on the model of Church schools. They saw their education as a way of becoming 'British Asians', rather than Asians from their 'home' country on the model of their parents.

People educated in the Western way are far more open to the way health care is done in the West. Shagufta, above, does not want to be Pakistani like her parents are, and wish her to be. She wants to be a British Asian. She understands her parent's attitude to health care but she fully accepts and is part of the British way of doing things. We are both in the same health care culture, even though she undoubtedly remains part of the occult and magic world that her parents inhabit.

- **Evolution**

In a sense, the cross-cultural problem is solving itself. First generation incomers, unless they are teenagers or younger, are unlikely to adapt to British culture to any significant extent. They will nearly always remain at heart a citizen of their country of origin. But their kids will be British and want to be British. This very frequently leads to a clash with their elders, who often can't see why their children are not growing up like the children in their home country. In a year or two, the children will want to stay in Britain and not go back to their home country. The crunch comes when the children go to school. Once this happens, the children will dig their heels in.

"I was in Pakistan for a month," said Rifat. "'That's it', I said to my mum. 'I'm never going back there!'"

These children grow up speaking English as well as their British friends. They are like Shagufta. She is completely British and understands how medical practice and all its ways works in Britain in a way her parents can never hope to. Young people like her can act as useful ambassadors to their own families, explaining how this incomprehensible country works.

- **Frequent Consultation**

For a number of reasons, consultations appear to be more frequent in areas where ethnic communities predominate. Unemployment can be one reason; Sharif came tirelessly every fortnight or so. There didn't seem to be much wrong. Then he got a job and I thought he had left town. No, he was at work and had stopped coming to the surgery. People came for social reasons, to meet their friends, parents brought their children to signal to their families that they were caring for them, or simply that they were anxious about them. People came because no one wanted to spend money on medicines that they could get free on prescription. A chemist told me "The over the counter sales on medicines in this street are zero!" This is a problem that has now been partially solved by the minor ailments scheme, but many of the factors that I have outlined above mean that the attendance rate will be high.

The family doctor finds herself in a position of extraordinary privilege. The Dr Rosinas of this country, if they can give the time and inclination, will make many good relationships. Accessibility, frequency of attendance, and confidentiality can be the foundation.

- **Trust**

People from abroad seem disposed to trust doctors more than those of our patients who were born and bred here. A very healthy change has occurred over the past few decades; we now regard our doctors and hospitals to be accountable and not above criticism. What a good thing this is, and how good for our professional standards, and how good for our self-image that we have been discovered to be fallible!

But ethnic minorities appear to be more trusting of nurses, doctors and health staff than native British people. This can be dangerous. This respect can lead to good relationships but we need to work overtime to ensure we are worthy of this trust. And we need to be honest when people's expectations are not met; honesty is a far better basis for a relationship than an inflated and unrealistic view of our competence.

- **The Moral High Ground**

I adopt a high moral tone without apology! What kind of a doctor or nurse, or physio or practice manager, are we and why are we in the business? The tradition of health care and medicine in Britain and Europe came out of a Judeo-Christian ethic where caring for the sick was seen as good in itself. Christian hospitals existed centuries before the NHS. Many of the great hospitals in Britain have Christian foundations.

I have mentioned Florence Nightingale and other great nurses; their work came out of this philosophy.

An essential part of this ethos was that it was not based on financial gain. It was based on the idea that caring for the sick was a good thing to do *in itself* because it was what Christ himself did. One might also argue that his healings were paid for at the point of delivery – there was certainly no waiting list and no appointment system, though you would doubtless have waited a long time to be seen on the day.

Another vital and essential aspect of this outlook was the special place for the 'fatherless and widows' and the poor. In past times, many of the sick were also poor and were unable to pay for care. They received it cheap or free.

One may quickly point out that there were many faults and many imperfections. People were abused as well as cared for. Nevertheless, the argument still holds.

A different ethos, such as the one I have outlined in Part 2 above, where private health care is the experience of many of our ethnic patients, and commerce is the unfettered driving force. This has virtually no moral motivation. It can never sustain a moral, corruption-free and kind health service. Those who work with ethnic minorities, refugees and immigrants are likely to be working with the poor. In many situations, the words are virtually synonymous. We have to have a reason for working in this environment. This is called a vocation or calling! I am suggesting that, as good health care workers, we will never be satisfied purely with a well-paid job. We need a calling; and most of us have one. Without this motivation, we will never go the second mile, a mile which is necessary to be good cross-cultural workers.

Looking at the sections above, I might hear you screaming, "But I simply don't have the time! It's just such hard work!"

Quite so; of course, we don't have the time and of course it is very hard work, especially today with the pressures on us as they are. But there remains a choice: am I going to make lots of money or am I going to provide a really good service? Of course, it isn't either/or. But there *is* a choice. I can tailor my practice to maximise profits, or I can settle for a little less and maximise service and satisfaction, both for patients, staff and myself. We have to accept the health service as it is and not be unrealistic about our expectations that it will improve. It is just not going to. Demands are becoming more strident, with the potential to intervene and treat increasing daily. The penalties for making mistakes are dire. Money is getting shorter… Get used to it!

- **The Professional High Ground**

The next step is to take cross-cultural communication seriously. Make it a sub -speciality in itself. Give it time and priority. Know that it produces results and gives increased patient satisfaction. It will boost your practice size, which may be the last thing you need. It is proven to give better clinical outcomes. And taking it seriously instead of begrudgingly will make it much more enjoyable for you and your colleagues.

- **The Anthropologist**

We can loosely define the anthropologist as one who studies people from other cultures. This is what we are going to learn to do. And we will find we are doing most of it already! Anthropology is a fascinating and totally rewarding subject. It helps to do a post graduate degree, or M. Phil, but that is not strictly necessary. Just read a few good basic anthropology text books and articles and put them in your work library.

- **Anthropological Methods:**

Location.
Get yourself where you can study your chosen people. Well, that's OK, you are there already. The bulk of your working day is spent with the people you are studying, your patient clientele. You don't have to go anywhere!

Make relationships.
You are doing this already. You are really working hard at making good relationships with your cross-cultural clientele. So the first two 'methods' you are already doing.

Watch.
Watch what people do, especially if they do things that British people would not do, or do differently in the same situation. Observe closely, especially if you don't have any idea what people are up to. Ask yourself, 'Why on earth are they doing this?' and a

whole area of ignorance and exciting inquiry will open up in front of you. If you don't know that you don't know you won't know to ask.

Why do the old women walk behind their husbands? Why do Sikh men wear those bangles? Why must this family bury grandpa pretty well on the same day he died and get really upset if it doesn't happen? People don't just do things for nothing. They do things for what, to them, are good reasons.

Ask questions.
People just love talking about their lives and will go on for hours. So you think people will take you for a real nosy parker and most intrusive? Not at all. If you have a good relationship with people, they will feel honoured that you are asking about them and their culture and what, to them, are their ordinary lives. Some areas that you might think are sensitive may turn out to not be so at all.

I wanted to learn about magic practices and their bearing on the cause and cure of illness. I started to ask mothers why they put those little black boxes round their children's necks. Was I told to mind my own business? No, they just couldn't stop talking. Many times you will not get the answer to the question you are asking, but you may get the answer to another question altogether. And don't be afraid to ask the same question many times to many different people; the more times you ask it, the more different answers you will get!

Don't try to keep people to the subject; this will shut them up. Let them ramble on. People will tell you stories, their experiences, traumas, family histories, how people got ill and how they got better – or didn't, how they escaped from burning buildings, crawled under or climbed over barbed wire fences in the 'Jungle' in Calais, and got to this country. They will tell of their mad uncles and other eccentric relatives, how their neighbour is involved in an affair, how their daughter was affected by the evil eye, how they are running a business on the side when they are not allowed to work. It is truly amazing what people will tell you if you are obviously interested, especially if you are their doctor! And all of it is important. People tend to talk in stories and personal experiences and that is exactly what you are looking for. Don't look for – or ask for – analysis or explanation. That is for you to do.

I started by using a carefully constructed questionnaire. It lasted until about 10 a.m. on day one then it got torn up.

Listen.
All this assumes that you are interested and are going to listen. But of course you have so little time. The waiting room is full and the practice manager has poked her head round the door to tell you that you have a rather full waiting room and will you please stop chatting and get a move on?

The 'new' consultation is about listening to people rather than obtaining answers to a prearranged set of questions, a mindset that inevitably leads to us interrupting our patients in full flow. What is the result? Unhappy patients!

But active – 'mindful' listening is a skill that we are all learning. It is no different from the kind of skills needed to conduct a successful consultation, only in cross-cultural work the information is of a slightly different kind. You are not trying to solve a puzzle or gather information that will lead to a diagnosis. You are just trying to learn about people. But the transition from one to the other may be easier said than done. Besides, a lot of your work will be done outside the consulting room.

Evolve a knowledge base.
You need to have some idea what you are looking for, but nothing too specific or you will miss something of great interest and importance! It needs to change as you learn about your people. This will allow you to build a picture in your mind of the kind of cultural features that will enable you to understand your clientele better. This will change all the time.

People are breathtakingly varied in their beliefs and habits and the more you learn, the more you will be surprised. You may have helpful little books about what Sikhs, Hindus and Muslims believe but the reality is for more complicated and far more interesting. You will also learn that people are not equally candid. I have found young people are generally less defensive about their culture and are much more likely to be honest. A western education has allowed younger people to be more insightful of their own culture.

Pool your knowledge. Make it important that you discuss cross-cultural issues, what you find difficult and what you have discovered, with staff and colleagues. Write something. Make this into an academic discipline in its own right and not just an 'add on'.

Let others know what you are doing. You are learning something special! And share all this with your colleagues.

Ask more Questions.
Never be tired of asking questions. You may well get a reputation for your inquisitiveness, and this will be to your benefit. People will realise that you are really interested in them. And keep adding to your knowledge base as a matter of habit.

- **Finding a Cultural Mentor**

You need someone on the inside to tell you trade secrets. You need a friend – or perhaps several friends – 'in the culture' who you can rely on to give honest answers. This is harder than it sounds – although, when I was in South Sudan I never found difficulty with this. When it came to calling a spade a spade, most people from South Sudan would put a Yorkshire person to shame.

You may not be so lucky, and some Middle Eastern cultures are very indirect. People will go round the houses to avoid being rude or confrontational and there may be a good deal of suspicion of 'foreigners', so it may be a while before you find someone. And which culture? I was very fortunate to work with a practice population of which about 40% originated from the same village in Kashmir. You might not be so lucky. In central Sheffield there are about forty different language groups. That doesn't necessarily mean forty separate cultures, but it does indicate great cultural variety – and huge communication challenges.

- **Get a Good Interpreter**

Language Line and other agencies are all very well, and are very useful when there is a proliferation of languages, or yet another new language on the block, but they are not to be compared with live interpreters.

The trouble with interpreters is the time that you allow for a consultation has to be doubled, hugely adding to the expense and use of time. The 'Mulberry clinic' in Sheffield, a dedicated health service for asylum seekers, holds to this principle and it works well, but at a cost in time double that taken by patients who did not require translation.

An 'embedded' translator can, of course, come from the community or communities that you are serving and act as an interpreter of culture and a way for community members to communicate with your practice.

Interpreters will have a way of communicating that is not your own cultural way and that will, in a practice, count for much more. A Sheffield practice where I was working experienced a rapid growth in its practice population from an East European country. Zofi comes from this culture and has her culture's expectation that the doctor will provide medicines and lots of them. On every occasion.

After some obviously hopeless attempts to explain the way doctors prescribe medicines in Britain, and after having seen a number of patients leaving with 'unhappy patient' signs firmly pinned between their shoulder blades, we sat down with our interpreter, a very insightful and intelligent young man from the same community. We discussed the matter in detail. He told us exactly what Zofi and her family and friends were expecting, which was hugely helpful. Then, rather than the doctor or nurse doing the talking, we worked out a way that he himself would explain things to the patient, in his own words, rather than ours; the way that we were trying to care for children and how medicines would fit into that. He would emphasise that if things did not get better we would see her or her children the next day or sooner, and that not giving medicines was not a sign that we were neglectful or didn't care.

This way, information and advice was coming from a person in their own culture and was immediately a little more acceptable. It also helped our patients negotiate the change from their health system at home to the one in Sheffield. It did not solve all the problems, but it was progress. We were very fortunate in our interpreter. We were very *un*fortunate in that he was employed only two days a week.

Your intelligent interpreter can help in another way. Learning the language of one or all of your ethnic groups is unrealistic except for enthusiasts. But your interpreter can teach you greetings and some simple polite phrases that go a long way to encourage your clientele that you are interested in them. It is a great mistake to learn to ask questions, even simple ones. This invites a stream of Serbian, Arabic, Kurdish or any another language, of which you understand not a word.

Your interpreter can, however, construct a brief questionnaire with possible answers. A TB sanatorium in the Middle East is in an Arabic speaking environment. On Fridays, large numbers of Bengali people attend the outpatient's department from the nearby garment factories where they have been working in sweatshop conditions. The hospital has found someone to compile a list of phrases which, though of limited use, represents a small amount of progress in communicating with these Asian people who know neither Arabic, English, Dutch, German or any of the other languages spoken in this multi-national hospital. It contributes to making them feel wanted and cared for, which is why they attend in the first place.

Our other big minority group in north Sheffield came from the subcontinent. We had two receptionists from the same community and both were happy to act as interpreters, frequently required as many women were poor in English, in spite of having spent many years in this country. But one receptionist was quite young and inexperienced, and there were situations where both found themselves rather uncomfortable, especially in cases where the patients were men. In addition, using receptionists in this way means taking them away from the reception desk, where they are doing important work. There is also the possibility that there will be a family relationship or other connection between them – known or unknown to you – which may cause embarrassment and reduce communication still further.

On the other hand, a receptionist or other member of staff from an immigrant ethnic group, will go home at the end of the day. There her family will question her or him on what goes on there in the practice and what is it like. They will act as an ambassador for you in the community, who will learn what you are like through the eyes of one of their own people.

Here are two suggested solutions with their drawbacks. Working across languages is always going to be expensive and time consuming if it is to be done at all effectively.

How about using relatives? This is at least cheap and is often resorted to but has many disadvantages. It is surprising how quickly the collective breaks down and people look for privacy. Children are inappropriate when it comes to obvious topics. Men may not like to talk about their man problems through their wife. Additionally, the relative is likely to add their slant on the matter and you will get the relatives perspective, not the patient's.

I have found that husbands do not make ideal interpreters for their wives when it comes to Asian couples. Men often take over. I asked a man to explain to his wife where we had got to in the consultation. "I will explain when we get home," he said.

Besides, women frequently behave in a subdued and rather obsequious way when in the presence of their husbands, as we have seen earlier. I have known women who could get by quite well in English but concealed the fact from their husbands, many of whom put every obstacle in the way of their wives learning the language.

"Just for goodness sake, *please* don't tell my husband I can speak English," one lady said.

- **Visits**

British general practice has a secret weapon that is found in few other countries – the home visit, or house call as it is sometimes referred to. It is said that you can't do good clinical work on home visits, and they are often held up as a great time waster. Well, home visits may not be good medicine but they are good anthropology! Besides, we are fortunate that we have health visitors and midwives who regularly visit at home.

Here you can see people in their own environment, and they are often more relaxed than in the surgery as they are on home territory. And people will talk. They will share their food with you and something of their lives as well if you let them. You will see relationships played out more naturally. You will observe old-young and male-female relationships at first hand. In many Asian homes, it is the young women who do nearly all the work. Looking at the older ladies lying on the couch or the sofa, you might come to some tentative conclusions as to why the older ladies tend to be overweight and a bit arthritic.

In a way, it is sad that the days of GPs doing their own night call is over; no one is pretending at 2 a.m. But you might find yourself working on the emergency service, which may possibly provide the same opportunities.

The social visit is also a marvellous opportunity to learn about the culture of your patients. Yes, it is time consuming, but you don't have to do many and it isn't necessarily the doctor or nurse who should be doing this. All your team are anthropologists!

The social visit is quite unlike either a medical visit or a visit to a British home. For a start, you don't need to be invited to an Asian home, so don't worry if no one has. In fact, in most Asian cultures you will never be invited. You are expected to just go! *You* ask *them* if you can call and they will be delighted.

The visit, or at any rate the first to a particular house or family, is a special occasion. Dress up. Take a large box of chocolates or a big bunch of flowers. In most cultures represented in the UK, people take their shoes off at the door. This is not just a habit but a way of showing respect to the home. So, take your shoes off at the door, even if your host tells you not to bother. In fact, the first visit is a formal one where you are honouring the home and family and they in turn are honouring you. You may be shown into a very ornately furnished guest room filled with lush furniture. This is the place of honour for guests and the rest of the house may be quite modest. You will be given food, which you absolutely must eat and enjoy (that isn't at all difficult). If you take your children, which is a great idea, you must warn them that they *must* eat and drink what is put in front of them. That said, children break down cultural barriers in minutes that take adults months or years to cross.

Of course, food and its customs will bring you into a whole new environment. A Sudanese friend kept piling food onto my plate while I remonstrated that I was absolutely full. He laughed and said that I had eaten everything on my plate like a well brought up English person is supposed to. In his culture, it would be a sign that I was still hungry and, as a good host, he should pile more and more onto my plate

"Just leave something on your plate," he laughed. "That will show you are full!"

Watch carefully to see what people do or don't do. If you do the same, you are not going too far wrong, but most people are very relaxed about cultural ignorance and they will just laugh tolerantly when you make the occasional blunder.

- **Teamwork**

None of this is individual. Whether we are in hospital or the community, we need to get the whole team geared towards doing cross-cultural work and alive to its opportunities. Having staff members from the people we are serving helps a lot. It is not so difficult to recruit receptionists and cleaners but nurses and doctors are further down the line. Still, having a couple of receptionists and certainly one or two cleaners is enormously helpful. They will give you lots of helpful advice, and as I have said, they will feed information back into the community that you are real people. They will tell stories at home of the extraordinary things you get up to but that you are really quite reasonable when they get to know you.

- **Conclusion**

I have tried to show that there are many factors that make your interaction with your 'ethnic' patients confusing and difficult, but in many cases these factors can be analysed and overcome. Understanding brings a degree of tolerance. I have tried to give a few words of advice to doctors from abroad who are trying to navigate this strange culture and funny rather cold people. I have tried to outline a number of factors that are on your side as you work with your ethnic patients that are going to make life a little more possible in the long run, if not just now, and briefly outlined some methods – not to call them techniques – that will help. I hope that I have encouraged you to see cross-cultural work as a vocation and a professional sub-speciality in its own right. I hope I have *not* succeeded in showing that cross-cultural work is easy. It isn't! Done properly, it is expensive in money, people and time. But I hope that the "unhappy patient" sign will slowly fall into disuse, and the "happy doctor" sign will come out of its drawer more and more often. Cross cultural practice done well is very worthwhile, it gives good outcomes, it produces happy patients and happy staff. And most of the time, it is very rewarding and great fun.

I end with a remark from the senior nurse in a practice in Sheffield, where the cross-cultural situation is exceptionally challenging. "The trouble is", she said, "This kind of work spoils you for anything else."

NOTES

[i] There is plenty of good literature about the good consultation. The gold standard is still *Skills for Communicating with Patients*. Jonathan Silverman, Suzanne Katz and Juliet Draper. Radcliffe Publishing. Reprinted 2008

[ii] *Long term Effects of Chronic Khat Use; Impaired Inhibitory Control.* Lorenzo S.Colzato, Manuel J. Ruiz, Wery P.M. van den Wildenberg, Maria Teresa Bajo and Bernhard Hommel. Frontiers in Psychology 2010;1;219. Published on line Jan 12th 2011. PMCID;PMC 3153824. Optimism, mild euphoria, excitation, talkativeness, increased energy and enhanced self esteem. (Breniesen et al 1990. Kalix 1996.) the half life is about 4 hours, depending on the amount of chewed khat. When the acute depletion, effects vanish users experience feelings of depletion, numbness, insomnia and depression, lack of energy and mental fatigue. Chronic (ie daily) use of khat is associated with increased blood pressure, development of gastro-intestinal tract problems, cytotoxic effects on liver and kidneys and keratotic lesions at the site of chewing. (al-Habori 2005)

[iii] FGM. The following sites may be useful.
https://www.womankind.org.uk/fgm/fgm-organisations-offering-advice-and-support

- Female genital mutilation (FGM) | NSPCC

*https://www.nspcc.org.uk/what-is-child-abuse/types-of-abuse/***female-genital-mutilation-fgm**

- Female Genital Mutilation Risk and Safeguarding

Nohttps://assets.publishing.service.gov.uk/government/uploads/system/... · PDF file

- Female genital mutilation (FGM) - NHS

*https://***www.nhs.uk***/conditions/***female-genital-mutilation**

Female genital mutilation (FGM) It's also known as female circumcision or cutting, and by other terms, such as sunna, gudniin, halalays, tahur, megrez and khitan, among others. FGM is usually carried out on young girls between infancy and the age of 15, most commonly before puberty starts.

[iv] *Communication with Relatives and Collusion in Palliative Care: A Cross-Cultural Perspective*, The Indian Journal of Palliative Care. Santosh K. Chaturvedi, Carmen G. Loiselle,and Prabha S. Chandra, 2009 Jan-Jun; 15(1): 2–9. doi: 10.4103/0973-1075.53485. this give a very helpful review of the interplay between patients, their relatives and doctors in communication in the area of death and dying in the cultural context of the subcontinent.
https://www.ncbi.nlm.nih.gov/pmc/articles/PMC2886207/

[v] Dr Debbie Hawker has very useful insights into post traumatic stress and advice on how it can be approached. *Debriefing Aid Workers and Missionaries: a Comprehensive Manual* 7th Edn. Dr Debbie Lovell-Hawker. People In Aid 2010
info@peopleinaid.org   www.peopleinaid.org)

[vi] For the concept of hot and cold cultures and other ideas in this chapter I am much indebted to Sarah Lanier *Foreign to Familiar*: *A Guide to Understanding Hot- And Cold-Climate Cultures.* Sarah A Lanier. McDougal Publishing 2000

[vii] In fact Sudanese English, like Indian English, has developed as a language with a life of its own with its own distinctive grammar and vocabulary, so perhaps the student was right!

Robin Fisher's email address is bartolemedelascasas@gmail.com